Intercollegiate Basic Surgical Skills course

Participant handbook

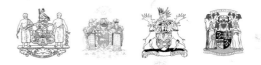

Fifth edition

This handbook was written by Mr Rory McCloy (Intercollegiate Basic Surgical Skills Development Tutor), Mr Bill Thomas (Chairman of the Intercollegiate Basic Surgical Skills Working Party) and Mr John Weston Underwood (Intercollegiate Basic Surgical Skills Quality Assurance Assessor).

Published by The Royal College of Surgeons of England
Registered Charity No. 212808

RCS Education
The Royal College of Surgeons of England
35–43 Lincoln's Inn Fields
London WC2A 3PE
Tel: 020 7869 6300
Fax: 020 7869 6320
Email: education@rcseng.ac.uk
Internet: www.rcseng.ac.uk

© The Royal College of Surgeons of England 2012
First edition 1996
Second edition 1998
Third edition 2002
Fourth edition 2007
Amended and reprinted fourth edition 2010
Fifth edition 2012

The intercollegiate working party would like to thank the following companies whose technical input and financial support has been invaluable in producing this fifth edition:
- Annex Art for their invaluable technical support of the Intercollegiate BSS courses
- ConvaTec for their help in developing the wound care section for the course handbook
- Covidien for their invaluable help in producing the Electrosurgery section for the course DVD and handbook
- Ethicon Products UK, who have provided materials and equipment for the delivery of the Intercollegiate BSS courses, and kindly supported the production of this fifth edition of the course.
- Limbs & Things for their invaluable technical support of the Intercollegiate BSS courses
- Mölnlycke for their ongoing financial support and commitment, and for the provision of Biogel gloves, for the Intercollegiate BSS courses

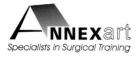
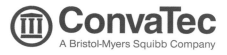
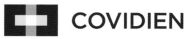
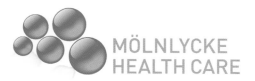
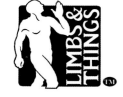

We are particularly grateful to Mr Peter Willson for developing the new electrosurgery section and Mr Nick Gillham for his orthopaedic input to the fifth edition.

Contents

Open surgery

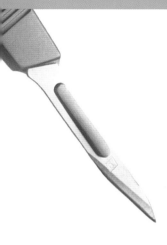

This section of the course is designed to teach you basic safe methods for performing simple surgical procedures, and to allow you to perform and practise them on the bench using prepared animal tissue, simulations and various jigs. We aim to provide you with an enjoyable hands-on experience and the opportunity of practising vital and fundamental techniques in an atmosphere that is less stressful than the operating theatre. The section aims to introduce you to some of the manipulative skills you will require in your career. Complex manoeuvres will need to be practised, preferably under critical observation, so that you do not acquire bad habits. The aim of this course is to help you acquire good habits early in your career, as it is so much harder to unlearn bad habits later in life. The techniques chosen for this course by all four surgical royal colleges are those which are simple and safe, but we make no claim that these are the only simple and safe techniques. An advantage of the British system of training is that you will work for many surgeons in the course of your training, each of whom will show you individually preferred techniques from which you will be able to select those that suit your needs best.

Knots

Knot tying is one of the most fundamental techniques in surgery and is often performed very badly. Take time to perfect your knot-tying technique as this will stand you in good stead for the rest of your career. Practise regularly with spare lengths of surgical thread.

General principles of knot tying include:

- The knot must be firm and unable to slip.
- The knot must be as small as possible to minimise foreign material.
- During tying do not 'saw' the material as this will weaken the thread.
- Do not damage the thread by grasping it with artery forceps or needle holders, except at the free end when using an instrument tie.
- Avoid excess tension during tying as this could damage the structure being ligated or even cause breakage of the thread.
- Avoid tearing the tissue that is being ligated by controlling tension at 'bedding down' of the knot, very carefully using the index finger or thumb as appropriate.

You will be taught and asked to demonstrate the following:

- the one-handed reef knot;
- an instrument-tied reef knot;
- the surgeon's knot;
- tying at depth.

When practising, tie your knots vertically over 'the wound', not down towards your lap. Standing up to tie knots is more representative of most surgical practices.

One-handed reef knot

A one-handed reef knot, properly thrown and laid, is the cornerstone of surgery. You will perform it with your left hand because your right hand may be holding the needle holder and also because it is easier to transfer your skills to your right hand later. Both throws are tied with the hands over the wound and are held horizontally. The one-handed reef knot consists of two throws, the coming down and the going up throw, performed alternately.

Coming down throw

If the short end of the thread leads away from you, perform the coming down throw first.

- Begin by bending the left elbow with the palm down and hand pointing towards you.
- Pick up the short end between the thumb and ring finger (Figure 3a).

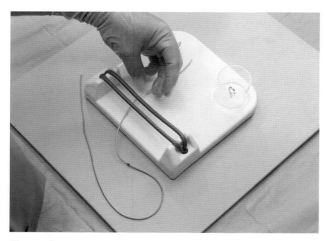

Figure 3a

- Now place the instrument over the thread again with the short end nearest to you (Figure 4e) and form a loop around the instrument by bringing the long end down and over and around the instrument (Figure 4f).

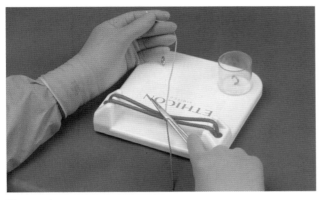

Figure 4e

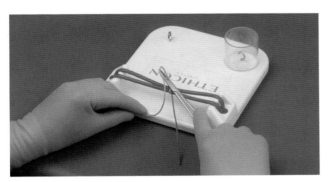

Figure 4f

- With the instrument through the loop grasp the short end again within the jaws of the instrument (Figure 4g).

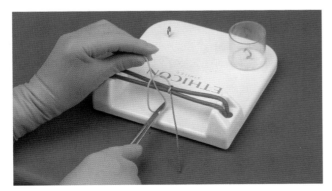

Figure 4g

- Pull through and cross the hands to complete the classical reef knot (Figure 4h).

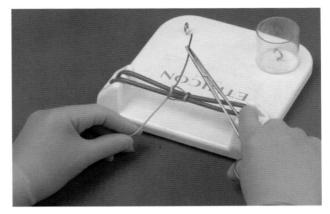

Figure 4h

The surgeon's knot

Sometimes we want a knot that is secure and will not slip between throws. To increase the friction in the first throw we can tie a double throw first and snug that down, and then return by a single throw. Although we do not have a very pretty looking knot, we have a very secure surgeon's knot.

- Begin in the same way as you did for the coming down throw of a single handed knot with your left hand, but hold the long end that is in your right hand as though it were about to perform a going up throw (Figure 5a).

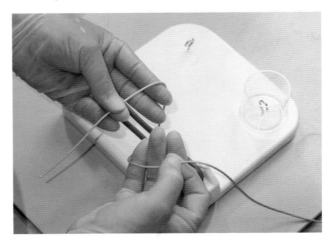

Figure 5a

- Separate the middle and ring fingers of the left hand.
- Form a loop by moving the right hand away from you over the middle and index fingers of the left hand so that your left index and middle fingers pass through the loop as usual (Figure 5b).

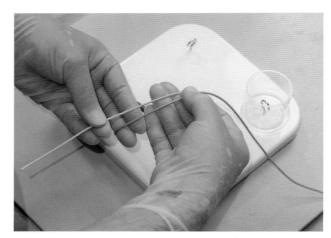

Figure 5d

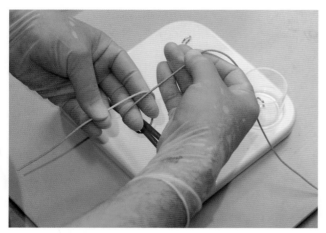

Figure 5b

- Then pass the middle ring and little fingers of the right hand through the same loop (Figure 5c) with the palm upwards above the left index finger (Figure 5d).

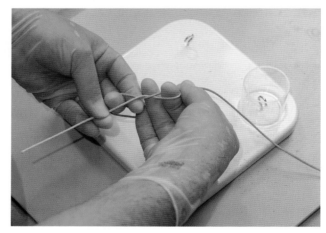

Figure 5e

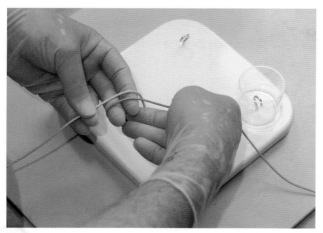

Figure 5c

- Bend both middle fingers under their respective ends of the thread and then straighten them so that the thread is on the back of each middle finger (Figure 5e).

- Using the index and middle fingers of the left hand, take the short end through the loop towards the left (Figure 5f) and at the same time take the long end through the loop towards the right using the middle and ring fingers of the right hand.
- Ensure the throw lies correctly by moving the left short end down towards you and the right long end away from you so that the hands cross (Figure 5g).
- Tighten appropriately (Figure 5h).
- Now perform a standard second single throw by doing a going up throw with the left hand (Figures 5i to 5k).

- When tying at depth, it is very important that the first throw does not come loose on the tissue whilst the second throw is being made and laid. For this reason it is common practice that the majority of ligatures at depth use a surgeon's knot on the first throw. This is best achieved by the single handed surgeon's knot technique (described above in Figures 6a–d).

Handling instruments

In order to achieve maximum potential from any surgical instrument it will need to be handled correctly and carefully.

The basic principles of all instrument handling include:

- safety;
- economy of movement;
- relaxed handling;
- avoiding awkward movements.

We shall demonstrate the handling of scissors, haemostats, needle holders, forceps and scalpel. Take every opportunity to practise correct handling using the whole range of surgical instruments.

Scissors

Scissors are designed for use in the right hand. There are two basic types of scissors, one for soft tissues and one for firmer tissues such as sutures.

- Insert the thumb and ring finger into the rings (or bows) of the scissors so that just the distal phalanges are within the rings (Figure 9). Any further advancement of the fingers will lead to clumsy handling and difficulty in extricating the fingers at speed.
- Use the index finger to steady the scissors by placing it over the joint.
- When cutting tissues or sutures, especially at depth, it often helps to steady the scissors over the index finger of the other hand (Figure 10).

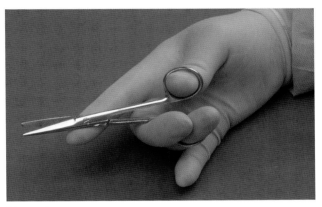
Figure 9

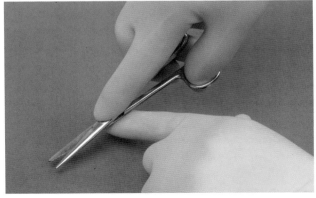
Figure 10

- Cut with the tips of the scissors for accuracy rather than using the crutch, which will run the risk of damaging tissues beyond the item being divided and will also diminish accuracy.

Haemostats (artery forceps)

Haemostats are designed primarily for use in the right hand. Haemostats may be curved or straight.

- Hold haemostats in a similar manner to scissors.
- Place on vessels using the tips of the jaws (the grip lessens towards the joint of the instrument).
- Secure position using the ratchet lock.
- Learn to release the haemostat using either hand. For the right hand, hold the forceps as normal, then gently further compress the handles and separate them in a plane at right angles to the plane of action of the joint. Control the forceps during this manoeuvre to prevent them from springing open in an uncontrolled manner. For the left hand, hold the forceps with the thumb and index finger grasping the distal ring and the ring finger resting on the under surface of the near ring (Figure 11). Gently compress the handles and separate them again at right angles to the plane of action, taking care to control the forceps as you do so.

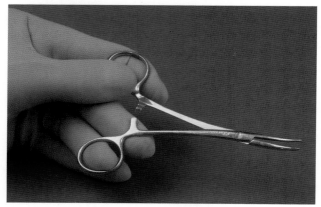

Figure 11

Needle holder

Needle holders are designed primarily for use in the right hand.

- A needle holder differs from a haemostat by way of the diamond-shaped milling of the 'teeth' which allows the shaft of a needle to be held securely at

any angle (Figure 12). The jaws may be lined with a harder metal than the steel of a needle shaft to prevent wear and damage to the instrument.

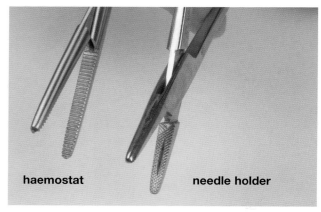

haemostat   needle holder

Figure 12

- Grasp the needle holders in a manner similar to scissors.
- Hold the needle in the tip of the jaws about two-thirds of the way along its circumference (Figure 13), never at its very delicate point and never too near the swaged eye (see Appendix A).

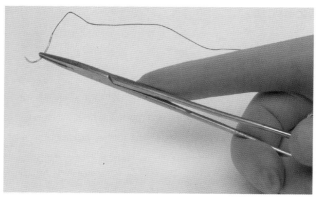

Figure 13

- Select the needle holder carefully. For delicate fine suturing use a fine short-handled needle holder and an appropriate needle. Suturing at depth requires a long-handled needle holder.

- Most needle holders incorporate a ratchet lock but some (eg Gilles) do not. Practise using different forms of needle holder to decide which is most applicable for your use.

- There are a wide variety of needle and suture materials available and their use will depend on the tissues being sutured and the nature of the anastomosis. For a full description of needles and suture materials see Appendix A and Appendix B.

- Practise the correct handling of each of the instruments (scissors, haemostats and needle holders) as demonstrated.

- Use the right hand first and then find out the limitations of using these instruments in the left hand.

Dissecting forceps

- Hold gently between thumb and fingers, with the middle finger playing the pivotal role (Figure 14).

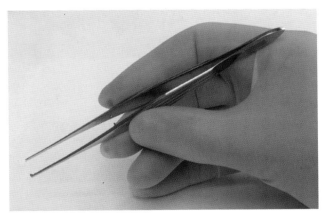

Figure 14

- Two main types of forceps are available: toothed for tougher tissue such as fascia or skin, and non-toothed (atraumatic) for delicate tissues such as bowel and vessels.

- Toothed forceps should not be used on tubular tissues as they can cause holes and potentially a leak.

- A third type of forceps are called Debakey (Figure 15) and have special longitudinal grooves which can grip tissues and needles.

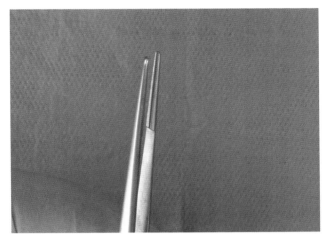

Figure 15

- Never crush tissues with the forceps but use them to hold or manipulate tissues with great care and gentleness.

The scalpel

- Handle with great care as the blades are very sharp. Never handle the blade directly. When attaching the blade to the handle the haemostat must not cross the cutting edge of the blade or else it will blunt or burr the blade. The angle at the base of the blade must be matched with the angled slot on the handle so that the blade can slide down the groove in the handle and lock in place (Figure 16). When removing the blade from the handle never point the tip down to the surgical drapes, as the patient beneath may be injured. The same applies to pointing the tip upwards or sideways because it may injure an assistant or yourself. Only remove the blade down onto the instrument trolley or into a suitable container.

- Practise attaching and detaching the blade using a haemostat.

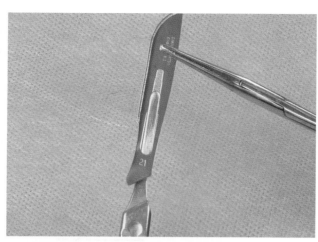

Figure 16

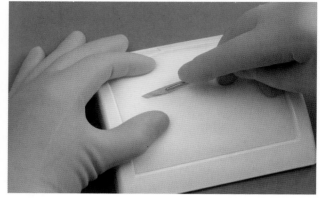

Figure 17

- For making a routine skin incision hold the scalpel in the palm of the hand, with your index finger guiding the blade. Keep the scalpel handle horizontal and the blade at right angles to the tissues to prevent shearing of the tissue edges. Then draw the whole length of the sharp blade, not just the point, over the tissues (Figure 17).

- For finer work the scalpel may be held like a pen, often steadying the hand by using the little finger as a fulcrum (Figure 18).

- Always pass the scalpel in a kidney dish. Never pass the scalpel point first across the table.

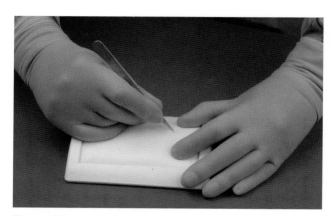

Figure 18

Basic principles

- Insert the needle at right angles to the tissue and gently advance through the tissue, avoiding shearing forces.
- As a rough rule of thumb, the distance from the edge of the wound should correspond to the thickness of the tissue, and successive sutures should be placed this distance apart (Figure 19).

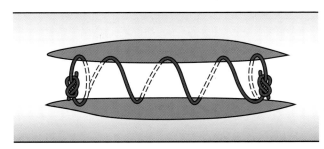

Figure 20a

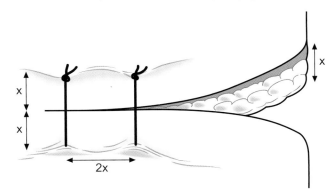

Figure 19

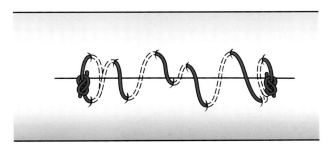

Figure 20b

- All sutures should be placed at right angles to the line of the wound at the same distance from the wound edge and the same distance apart to ensure equal tension down the wound length. The only situation where this should not apply is when suturing fascia or aponeuroses, when the sutures should be placed at varying distances from the wound edge to prevent the fibres parting (Figures 20a and 20b).
- For closing long wounds with interrupted sutures, it is advisable to place the first stitch in the middle of the wound, and subsequent stitches half way along that length, and so on.

- No suture should be tied under too much tension otherwise subsequent oedema of the wound may cause the sutures to cut out or to cause ischaemia of the wound edge and delayed healing.
- In most cases it is advisable to go through only one edge of the tissues at a time but, if the edges lie in very close proximity and accuracy can be ensured, it is permissible to go through both edges at the same time.
- The edges of elliptical wounds, following lesion excision, may be undermined to help closure. However, the length of the wound will need to be approximately three times the width of the wound if closure is to be safe and not under too much

tension. Skin hooks may be useful to display the wound.

Forms of suturing

You will be taught and asked to demonstrate the following types of suturing:

- interrupted sutures;
- continuous sutures (including the art of 'following');
- mattress sutures;
- subcuticular sutures;
- inverting and everting techniques.

Interrupted sutures (Figure 21)

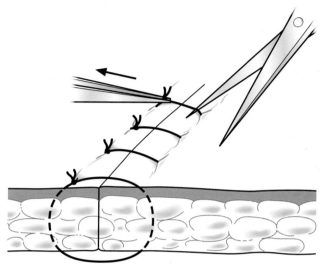

Figure 22a

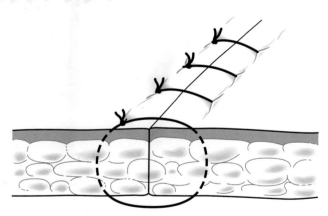

Figure 21

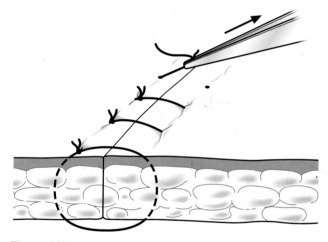

Figure 22b

- Place these carefully at right angles to the wound edges.
- Tie a careful reef knot and lay it to one side of the wound.
- Cut suture ends about 0.5 cm long to allow enough length for grasping when removing.
- When removing sutures, cut flush with the tissue surface so that the exposed length of the suture (which may be contaminated) does not have to pass through the tissues (Figures 22a and 22b).

Continuous sutures (Figure 23)

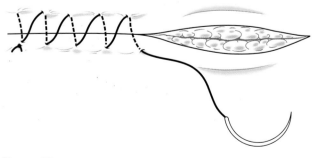

Figure 23

- Place a single suture and tie, but only cut the short end of the suture.
- Continue to place sutures along the length of the wound. Tension is determined by the surgeon and maintained at that tension by the assistant when the suture is passed to them.
- Take care not to 'purse-string' the wound by using too much tension.
- Take care not to produce too much tension by using a suture that is too short.
- Secure the suture at the end of the wound by a further reef knot.

Mattress sutures

- Mattress sutures may be either vertical (Figures 24a and 25a) or horizontal (Figures 24b and 25b).
- They may be useful for ensuring either eversion (Figures 24a and 24b) or inversion (Figures 25a and 25b) of a wound edge.

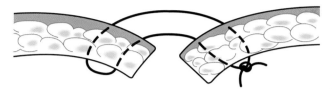

Figure 25a

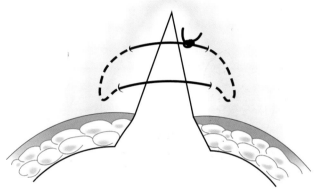

Figure 25b

Subcuticular sutures (Figure 26)

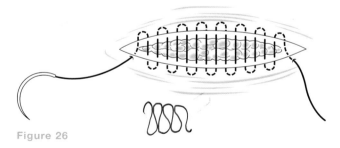

Figure 26

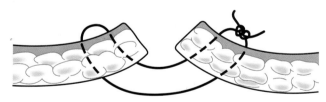

Figure 24a

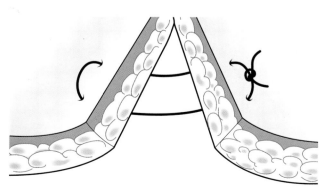

Figure 24b

- Subcuticular sutures are a snake-like continuous suture in the horizontal plane of the skin as opposed to a vertical spiral plane of the previous sutures.
- This technique may be used with absorbable or non-absorbable sutures.
- Small bites are taken of the subcuticular tissues on alternate sides of the wound, which are then pulled carefully together.

See *Appendices B* and *C* for further information on needles and suture materials.

Handling tissues

Tissue dissection

There are two methods of tissue dissection; sharp and blunt.

- With sharp dissection you use scissors or a knife; taking great care over the tissues to make sure you don't damage neighbouring structures.
- Then start developing a plane by sharp dissection. Having started to do some sharp dissection (Figure 27).

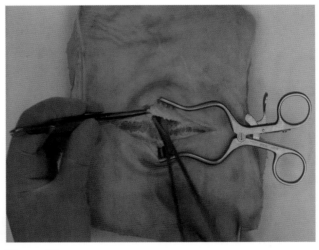

Figure 28

- This way you are not going to damage any structure because you're doing it gently by blunt dissection with your finger (Figure 29).

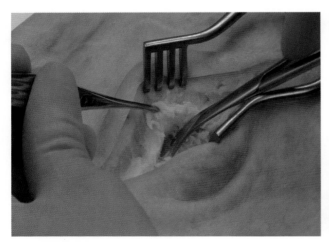

Figure 27

- You may find it useful to turn the scissors the other way up and just gently open the blades, teasing the tissues apart (Figure 28).
- It may be appropriate to ask your assistant to insert a retractor or two, to help your exposure and then there is a time when finger dissection helps develop the plane even further.

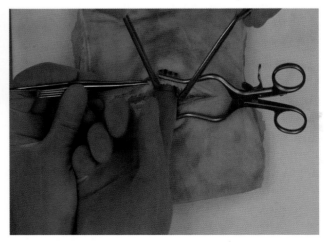

Figure 29

- Good tissue dissection often requires all three approaches.

Local anaesthetic technique

Safe doses of lignocaine

- The maximum safe dose of lignocaine is 3 mg/kg (6 mg/kg with adrenaline).
- The standard ampoule of 1% lignocaine contains 10 mg/ml.
- Therefore, the usual safe total volume of 1% lignocaine to be infiltrated in a 70 kg patient is 21 ml.

- Before excising a skin lesion you can practise the administration of local anaesthetic to the planned area of excision (best marked out with a suitable pen).
- There are two techniques. The first 'static' technique involves inserting the needle at the site of instillation and aspirating to make sure the tip is not in a blood vessel – no 'flash-back' of blood. It is then safe to inject the local anaesthetic as inadvertent intravenous injection could lead to cardiac dysrhythmias (Figure 30).

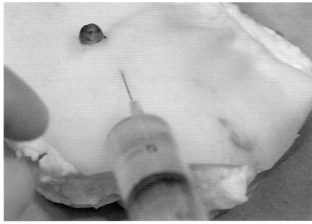

Figure 30

- The second technique involves continuous movement of the needle through the tissues while injecting the local anaesthetic. Any passage through a blood vessel would be transient and intravenous injection of any significant volume would not occur.

- It is kinder to start with a fine-bore needle until the initial area has been anaesthetised and then change to a longer, large-bore needle for infiltration of the planned surgical field.
- Check the planned area of incision has been successfully anaesthetised by gently touching with the tip of the scalpel blade and asking the patient if there is any sensation, before making a full incision.

Excision of skin lesion

- Identify the skin lesion for excision and, assuming it to be benign, leave a 1-mm margin either side. Estimate the planned width. Then calculate the length of the elliptical excision as three times the width. This is the minimum width to length ratio for a cosmetic closure without undue tension (Figure 31).

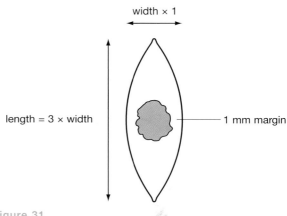

Figure 31

- If the area allows, then a 1 to 4 width to length ratio is even better.
- You can use a suitable skin marker to help plan the area and ensure the correct field for excision is infiltrated with local anaesthetic.
- After local anaesthesia has been achieved, excise an ellipse of skin, complete with lesion, and a portion of subcutaneous tissue shaped like the hull of a

boat (Figure 32) – this helps the skin to be closed without tension and avoids any risk of leaving part of the lesion deep to the skin if it had penetrated the dermis.

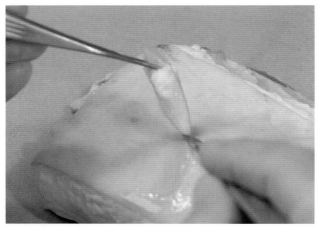

Figure 32

- Close the skin with interrupted vertical mattress sutures starting at alternate ends and working towards the centre.

Excision of sebaceous cyst

- Identify the 'sebaceous cyst' in your model.
- Plan a linear incision over the 'roof' of the cyst which is no longer than the diameter of the cyst (Figure 33). If a 'punctum' is visible, include this in your incision by taking a very narrow ellipse of skin (Figure 34).

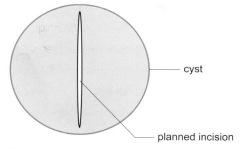

Figure 33

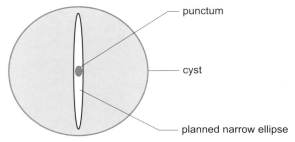

Figure 34

- Work carefully through the subcutaneous tissues, using a combination of blunt and sharp dissection techniques, until the 'capsule' of the cyst is reached. Then carefully work round all sides staying close to the capsule – avoid puncturing the cyst!
- Close the skin with either interrupted simple sutures or a subcuticular suture.

Ligation/Transfixion

Three methods of securing haemostasis by ligation will be demonstrated using vessels in small bowel mesentery.

Pedicle transfixation

This technique is used for fatty or bulky pedicles where a vessel could retract from the surrounding tie and cause frank haemorrhage or a haematoma in the tissues of the pedicle.

- Divide a large pedicle of tissue between haemostats.
- Using a round-bodied needle, transfix the pedicle with the suture just below (on the 'upstream' side) of the haemostat, about one-third of the way along the pedicle, and pull the suture through (Figure 35).
- Tie the first throw of a reef knot round the smaller end of the pedicle, tighten the throw, then pass the free end of the thread around the far side of the pedicle and tie another throw of the reef knot while the assistant gradually releases the tissues from the clip to allow them to bunch up and the suture to tighten. Finally, throw two more alternate throws of a reef knot.

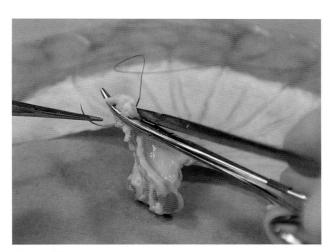

Figure 35

Continuity ligation

This technique is often used for larger vessels where a divided and untied vessel (if lost from the haemostat or tie as the knot is secured) could have disastrous consequences.

- Carefully dissect out a single vessel in the mesentery by dividing the peritoneum over it and isolating a length of vessel on its own.
- If possible, do not go right through the peritoneum on the other side of the mesentery.
- Pass ligature threads under the vessel by means of haemostats and ligate at either end of the isolated length of vessel.
- Divide the vessel between the two ligatures (Figure 36) and cut the excess suture material.

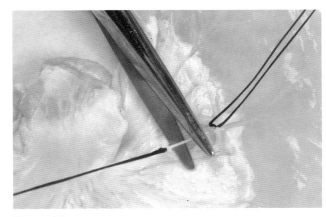

Figure 36

Clip ligation

This is the commonest form of vessel tie.

- Isolate a pedicle or leash of vessels and place a haemostat at either end.
- Divide the vessels between the haemostats.
- Ligate the vessels in each haemostat with a three-throw reef knot (Figure 37), taking care to tighten the knot with equally opposing forces (at 180°) which do not tug at, or displace, the vessel and clip. If curved haemostats are used it is easier to secure the tie if the curve of the clip is away from the knot.

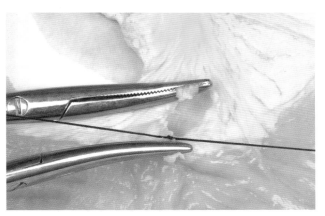

Figure 37

Bowel anastomosis

The basic principles of bowel anastomosis will be demonstrated using a small bowel anastomosis.

The essentials for any bowel anastomosis are:

- no tension;
- good blood supply (pulsating mesenteric vessels);
- accurate apposition;
- impeccable and accurate suture technique.

Many surgeons would prefer a single layer extramucosal suture (Figure 38). If you are suturing animal or paediatric tissues they may be too thin to allow an extramucosal suture, and an all-layers suture is acceptable.

The exercise will be performed as an end-to-end anastomosis on mobile small bowel that can be turned to reveal the posterior wall. Interrupted sutures will be placed and hand ties used to practice knotting techniques.

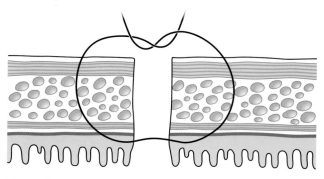

Figure 38

End-to-end anastomosis – interrupted suture

- Assume resection of a lesion.
- Line up the ends of the bowel. In operative circumstances non-crushing bowel clamps may be used to prevent spillage.
- Use 3/0 absorbable suture material with an atraumatic round-bodied needle.
- Insert stay sutures at the mesenteric and antimesenteric borders. Do not tie them but place in haemostats.
- Starting from the mesenteric aspect, place interrupted sutures along the anterior wall of the bowel approximately 4–5 mm apart and hand tie three-throw reef knots as they are placed. On completion, tie both stay sutures, but do not cut and replace in haemostats.
- Pass the mesenteric stay suture under bowel to emerge at the antimesenteric side. At the same time, draw the antimesenteric stay suture over the bowel in the opposite direction, which will reverse the bowel so the posterior wall will now lie anteriorly.
- Suture the 'new' front wall in a similar manner using interrupted sutures, taking care that the angles are adequately sutured.
- On completion, return the stay sutures to their original

position (Figure 39), then cut them and inspect the anastomosis.

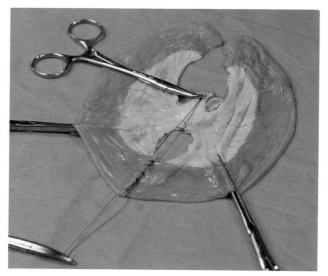

Figure 39

- In normal situations the mesenteric defect must be closed, taking care not to damage the mesenteric vessels.
- The anastomosis should then be tested for leaks, with fluid injected into the lumen under moderate pressure.
- In the exercise situation, cut out the anastomosis and then open it up and inspect it from the inside as well as the outside.

Tendon repair

Tendon surgery, particularly in the flexor tendon sheath in the hand, demands high surgical expertise and is beyond the remit of surgeons at ST1 level. Rehearsing the technique, however, is of considerable value in developing surgical competence. Crushing, or other forms of surgical trauma, will provoke fibrous tissue reaction and lead to tenodesis. Improper or inadequate tension of the sutures will leave voids and cause failure of the repair. This will be tested by distracting the repaired ends.

- The trotter of the pig includes a human-like arrangement of the superficialis and profundus tendons. Display a main profundus tendon and cut it transversely with a knife.
- At all times handle the tendon with care as forceps may cause crushing.
- The tendon is usually bean-shaped in cross-section (Figure 40). Using 4/0 braided polyester, install the sutures in the proximal tendon end first, starting at the cut end. The entry suture should pass through the middle of one half of the sectioned tendon, and follow a path parallel to the collagen fibres to 1.5 cm, or approximately the diameter of the tendon, and then exit. Refer to the diagram for a Kessler suture (Figure 41).

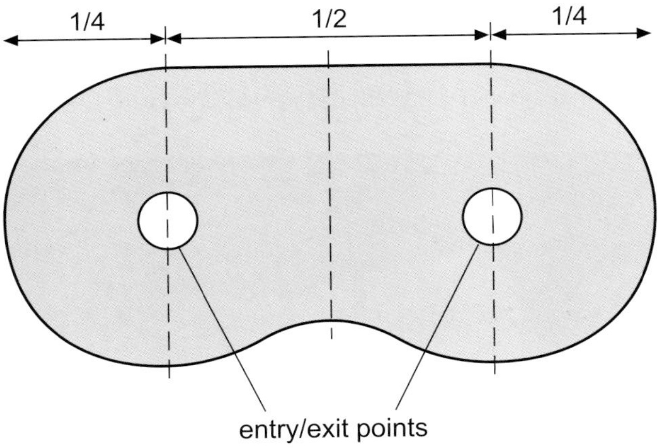

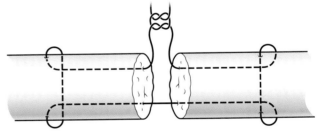

- The transverse component of the suture now passes a loop back just distal to the exit point and through the central half of the tendon. Now make the reciprocal longitudinal suture pass, exiting accurately in the middle of the second tendon half. Repeated misjudged needle placement is poor technique.
- Repeat the procedure into the distal end, having checked carefully the orientation of the tendon so that it will match the proximal end when the suture is tightened. Having placed the sutures in a satisfactory position, reduce the tendon accurately using the hypodermic needles and transfix in the reduced position. Tighten the suture, which will then leave the tail and needle ends of the suture to be tied and triple-knotted so that the knot is buried within the cut tendon end (Figure 42).

Figure 42

- Remove the transfixing hypodermic needles and apply tension to the tendon to ensure that the suture is performing adequately. If separation occurs the suture must be repeated.
- Insert the running stitch using 4/0 nylon (Figure 43). Insert the needle into the paratenon approximately 2 mm away from the cut edge. Put a clip on the end. Do not over-tighten. Each bite of the running suture should be at a separation of approximately 2 mm. Rotate the tendon using the suture until the complete running suture is in position. Tie off to the original starting suture at the end.

1/4   1/2   1/4

entry/exit points

Figure 40

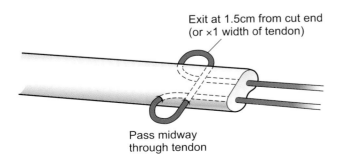

Exit at 1.5cm from cut end
(or ×1 width of tendon)

Pass midway
through tendon

Figure 41

Running 4/0 nylon

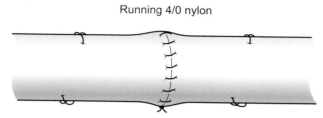

Figure 43

Abdominal incision, drain placement and closure

- The model representing the abdominal wall consists of layers of material that simulate the skin, subcutaneous tissues, linea alba and peritoneum. The layers are stretched over an inflated balloon which represents distended loops of bowel within the abdominal cavity. The aim of the exercise is to enter the peritoneal cavity without damaging the inflated balloon, to place and secure an abdominal drain, and to close the abdominal wall – all without bursting the balloon!
- Make a midline incision in the simulated abdominal wall skin (Figure 44a).

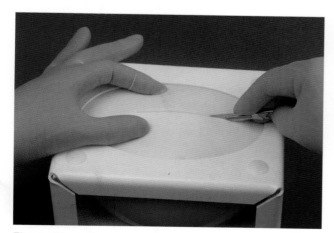

Figure 44a

- Expose the simulated linea alba and carefully incise with the 'belly' of a large scalpel blade.

- Then expose the simulated peritoneum and lift up using haemostats placed perpendicular to the line of the incision (Figure 44b).

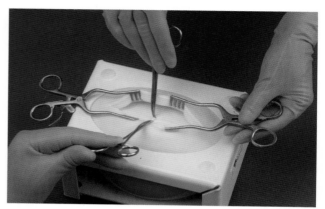

Figure 44b

- Incise the peritoneum carefully, using the 'belly' of a large scalpel blade, ensuring there is no damage to the underlying balloon (Figure 44c).

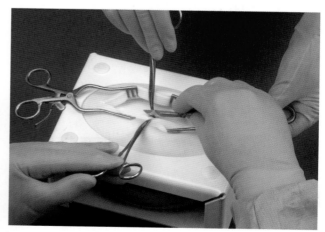

Figure 44c

- Enlarge the incision using scissors until the incision is adequate for whatever procedure is intended (Figure 44d). The peritoneal incision should be as long as the skin incision, otherwise the patient suffers a longer scar than the size of the access to the abdominal cavity. It is particularly easy to make this mistake in obese patients.

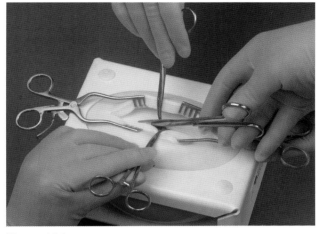

Figure 44d

- Before you close the abdominal wall you will need to place an abdominal drain. Make a small skin incision, lateral to the end of the wound, no larger than the diameter of the drain. Place a large clip from outside to inside, pointing through the fascia, towards your hand, which should be placed within the abdomen at the anticipated site of the clip entry in order to protect the bowel and internal organs from injury (Figure 45).

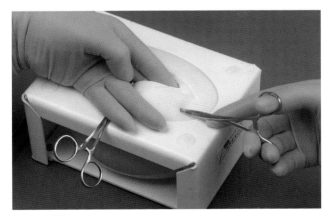

Figure 45

- Pull the drain through from inside to out (Figure 46). Once the drain has been placed at the correct site

and depth of insertion, secure it with a drain stitch to prevent accidental removal or displacement as the abdomen is closed. This is one of the rare occasions when a silk suture may still be used – it grips the drain securely and looks different from other skin sutures. Loosely tie a skin suture at the base of the drain and then pass the suture from side to side with single throws of a knot, working your way up 2 or 3 cm of drain, taking care not to constrict the drain lumen while still gripping the drain securely. Finish off with a three-throw reef knot and cut the ends long (Figure 47).

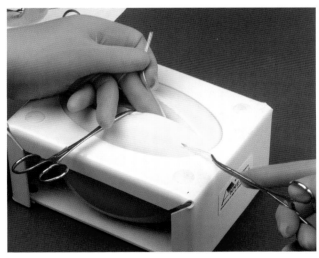

Figure 46

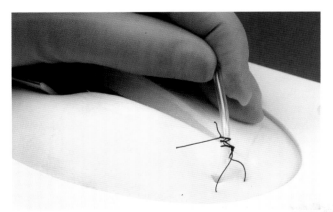

Figure 47

- Proceed to close the incision. Currently many surgeons use a blunt needle for this procedure (Figure 48), to minimise the risk of needlestick injuries, and a loop suture.

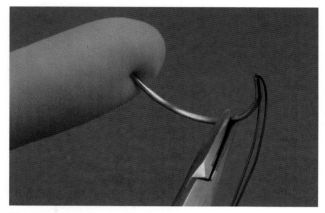

Figure 48

- The length of the suture should be four times that of the incision in order to ensure that there is enough suture material for 1-cm bites placed less than 1 cm apart (Figure 49). The suture should not be pulled too tight as this could result in tissue necrosis. If the suture length is not adequate, a further suture can be inserted starting at the other end of the incision.

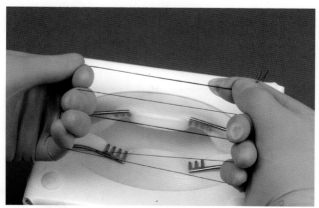

Figure 49

- When a loop suture is used the initial knot can be simply achieved by passing the needle through the loop and pulling tight (Figure 50).

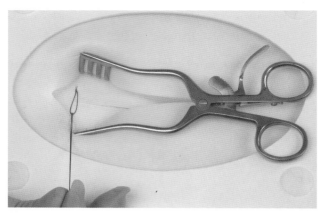

Figure 50

- Close the entire wound with this continuous suture, always ensuring that no loop of bowel or tissue is caught up by the suture material.
- Tie the suture material at the end of the closure using an Aberdeen knot. The complete closure should then be inspected.

The Aberdeen knot

- This knot is useful when, having finished a continuous suture, you are left with a loop and a free end (Figure 51a).

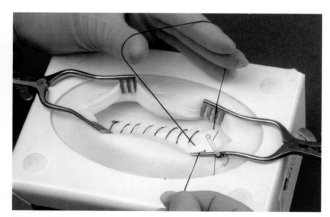

Figure 51a

- Display the loop between the index finger and thumb of your left hand. Grasp the strands going to the needle with the middle finger of the left hand through the loop (Figure 51b). Then by pulling it through with the index, middle and ring fingers (some surgeons also include their little finger) of the left hand and releasing the right-hand thread, eliminate the old loop (Figure 51c).

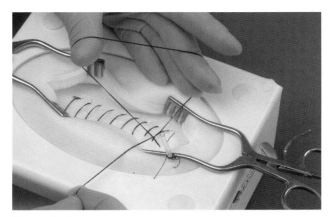

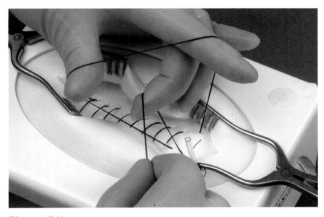

Figure 51b

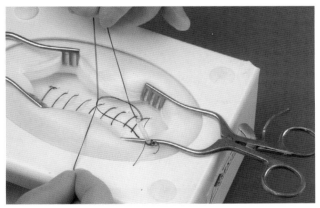

Figure 51e

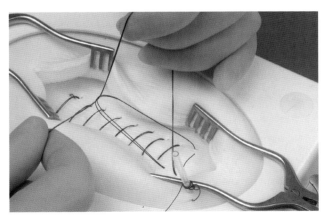

Figure 51c

- Once again a new loop is displayed between thumb and fingers (Figure 51d). Repeat the whole process using a type of 'see-saw' movement to pull it tight (Figure 51e).
- Repeat the whole process at least five times.
- Finally, pass the free end with the needle through the loop (Figure 51f) and tighten down.

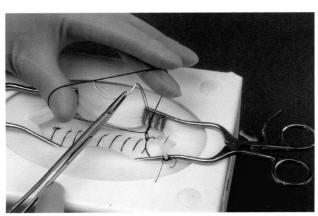

Figure 51f

In the abdominal wall exercise we do not want the cut ends of a large-gauge suture to 'prick' the skin from inside the wound and lead to postoperative discomfort. Under these circumstances the knot and the free end can be buried under the tissues by passing the needle back through the wound under several loops of the running suture (Figure 51g), taking care to stay within the layers of the abdominal wall and not catch the peritoneum or intra-abdominal contents beneath. Then cut the suture flush (Figure 51h).

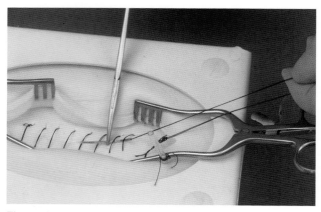

Figure 51g

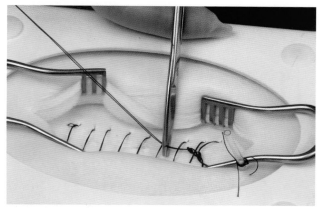

Figure 51h

Vein patch

Vessels need to be handled in a very different manner from bowel. Extreme gentleness in handling is required, and,

whenever possible, a vessel should be manipulated by grasping the peri-arterial or adventitial tissues only. When direct manipulation is unavoidable, arterial wall should never be grasped between forceps for fear of injury to the intima or even a full-thickness tear. Two methods for atraumatic handling of vessel walls may be used, either using the tips of closed Debakey (or dissecting) forceps to gently open the arteriotomy (Figure 52) or using the suture material to be used for the anastomosis to retract the arterial wall.

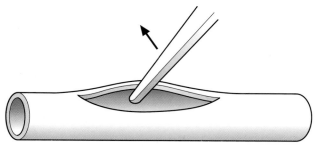

Figure 52

When suturing arterial wall it is advisable for the needle to pass from inside to out (ie from intima to adventitia) to fix any atherosclerotic plaques and prevent the formation of intimal flaps, which may lead to dissection, embolisation or thrombosis.

Non-absorbable, monofilament suture material that moves smoothly through the vessel wall is required. These suture materials require a careful knot technique and several throws to prevent the knot unravelling (most vascular surgeons recommend six or seven throws). Do not damage the suture material by gripping it with dissecting forceps, the needle holder, or a haemostat as this can lead to fracture. For the same reason, all knots need to be hand tied and the haemostat jaws covered with rubber or portex tubing (rubber-shod) to cushion the rough milling on the instrument.

Fine, accurate, watertight sutures need to be inserted at even tension when suturing vessels. Always insert the needle at right angles to the wall and pass it through the wall with several short 'pushes' that allow the needle to travel on the arc of its own circle, thus not splitting or tearing the delicate wall.

The finer the vessel, the finer the sutures required and the smaller the bites taken. Therefore, aortic sutures need large bites, while femoral sutures require fine bites. Distal anastomoses are often facilitated by operating 'loupes' – glasses that magnify the image by two to four times.

A smooth internal suture line is essential otherwise platelet aggregates will collect and compromise the anastomosis. The suture line needs to be everted to result in good intimal apposition, unlike a bowel anastomosis in which the suture line tends to be inverted.

A vein patch is the safest way to close an arteriotomy if there is the slightest suspicion that direct closure will produce narrowing.

- Make a longitudinal elliptical arteriotomy about 3 cm long in the vessel provided. Then cut one end of an elliptical patch in the simulated vein patch or prosthetic material provided. Leave the other end of the patch long and unshaped at this stage. The redundant portion can be used to handle the patch without damaging intima which will be in contact with flowing blood in vivo.
- Using a double-ended 4/0 monofilament polypropylene suture, insert an initial stitch from outside to inside at the shaped end of the patch and then pass it inside to outside through the apex of your arteriotomy (Figure 53). Then repeat this by using the needle on the other end of the suture and place it close to the other suture, again passing in through the patch and out through the artery. Tie the suture on the outside of the vessel and anchor one end in a rubber-shod haemostat.
- Take the free end of the suture and work down the far side of the arteriotomy. Insert continuous stitches using fine bites while holding the redundant portion of the patch with your forceps (Figure 54). It is not

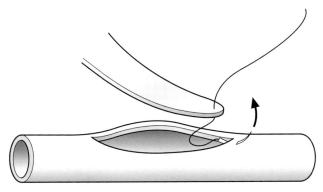

Figure 53

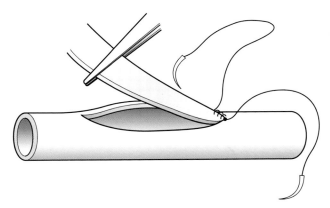

Figure 54

advisable to suture both vein patch and arterial walls with a single traverse of the needle unless you are experienced. Suture the two walls separately.

- When you near the heel of the arteriotomy, cut the patch to length transversely and then shape into an ellipse. Continue around the apex and place two or three sutures along the proximal wall.
- Now move back to your original suture and continue along the proximal wall until you meet the original suture. Flush inflow and outflow vessels before tying the two sutures at this point.
- At the end of the procedure cut open the back of the artery and observe the anastomosis from within the lumen. There should be no roughness and no irregularity or inversion of the suture line.

Debriding an infected wound

Frank pus requires drainage, and radiological-guided techniques may be appropriate depending on the anatomical situation. Surgical techniques remain the mainstay of treatment and the principles are adequate incision, evacuation of the pus, and debridement or curettage of the cavity. The cavity is best kept open to allow drainage by placing a light dressing in the wound. Traditionally surgeons have used gauze, but recent advances in dressing technology mean that there are now better alternatives available. For example, you may wish to consider using a silver impregnated Hydrofiber™ dressing with microbiocidal activity which can help control the wound bioburden, in conjunction with any systemic antibiotic therapy indicated by the clinical condition of your patient.

- Palpate the model for the most fluctuant area and incise with a large scalpel. Deepen the incision until the abscess cavity is penetrated and express the free pus. In the clinical situation a specimen would be taken for microbiology at this stage.
- Extend the wound to get adequate access to the cavity. A cruciate incision is preferred for abscessess around the perineum or abdomen as it is less likely to close as quickly as a linear incision (Figure 55a). However, a cruciate wound should be avoided in cosmetically sensitive areas such as neck and breast.

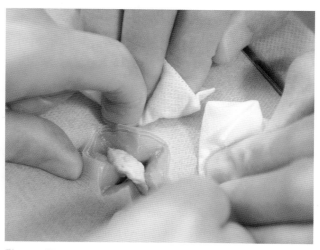

Figure 55a

- Place an opened swab over your index finger and sweep it around the cavity (Figure 55b). This scouring action removes the inflammatory debris and remaining pus and is an alternative to a curette or spoon instrument (which if roughly used can cause damage by penetrating the wall of the abscess).

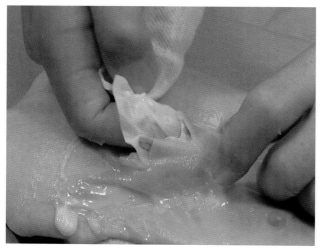

Figure 55b

- Once the cavity has been cleared of free and loose debris, simply place a loose gauze into it.

Debriding a traumatic wound

The primary care of a contaminated wound is pivotal for its subsequent healing. It is frequently undertaken imperfectly. Secondary procedures, once inflammation and scarring are established, may result in chronic disability. Six components to traumatic wound management are to be considered:

- wound toilet and irrigation;
- inspection of the wound;
- deep palpation of the wound;
- excision of dead or contaminated tissue;
- establishment of adequate drainage;
- dressing of the wound for later inspection.

In the clinical setting it may be prudent to select an alginate dressing with haemostatic properties for this type of wound. Alternatively you might consider using a modern dressing that can manage exudate and optimise wound bed conditions. Usually, this type of wound will be re-inspected at 48 to 96 hours post surgery when further excision and possibly skin grafting may be appropriate.

- You will be supplied with a leg either from a lamb or a large turkey in which there is a simulated traumatic contaminated wound.
- Clean the wound with water. Normal irrigant and antiseptics are water-based rather than spirit-based when dealing with open tissues. Cleansing should be done both by irrigation and with a swab (Figure 56a).

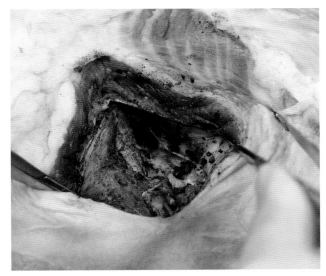

Figure 56b

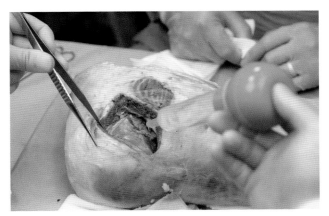

Figure 56a

- Initial inspection should identify gross contaminants and foreign material (Figure 56b). The wound will have simulated glass or pebbles embedded within. It is essential that you remove all of these (Figure 56c).
- Following the initial inspection, make a methodical detailed examination using forceps and retraction. Work methodically, for example clockwise, so that no component of the wound is left unexamined. Look out for and identify any structural anatomy including nerves, vessels and tendons. You may be asked to demonstrate these.
- Palpate to reveal tracts that might otherwise be overlooked. Again you should undertake this

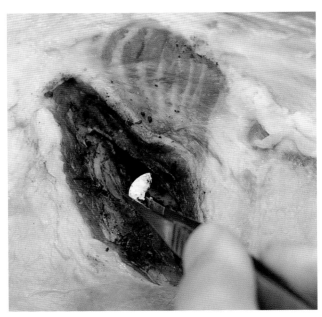

Figure 56c

methodically and use it as a further opportunity to examine every aspect of the wound. Foreign material may be felt by fingertip, but be careful of sharp glass or bone spicules. Where a large overhang is present, it is wise to extend the wound to permit adequate toilet.

- Excise all 'dead' tissue, including devitalised bone where necessary, cutting back to healthy muscle (Figure 56d). There is an appropriate amount of excision to be undertaken, but too little is worse than too much. Open up all cavities.
- Any cavity or sump must be adequately drained and may justify the use of a dependent drain. This model does not require drainage.
- Finally wash the wound, which is not closed. In this exercise a gauze is applied lightly to the cavity to allow tissue fluids to drain from the wound freely.

See *Appendix D* for further information on wound management.

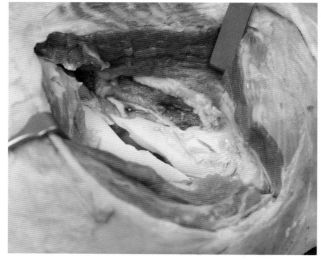

Figure 56d

The generation of heat

Heat has been used by surgeons for centuries to control haemorrhage. Historically, for example, hot cautery irons and tourniquets were used in battlefield and amputation surgery to seal wounds. These cautery techniques transferred heat to tissue by conduction but resulted in significant collateral tissue necrosis.

Modern cautery devices use a direct current to heat a resistor, usually in the form of a wire, which the surgeon applies to the area to be cauterised. They have a minimal role in 21st century surgery.

In contrast the art and science of electrosurgery (surgical diathermy[1]) is the conversion of electrical current into clinically useable heat. The patient is made part of an electrical circuit and by the use of different current types and surgical techniques various type of cutting and haemostasis are possible.

Basic Principles of Electrosurgery

Electrosurgical currents are delivered to patients in one of two ways; monopolar and bipolar.

Monopolar currents incorporate a large part of a patient in the circuit (Figure 57). Current passes between a surgical

---

[1]The term electrosurgery has been used throughout this section as the international term for the technique termed diathermy in the UK. The term diathermy when used in other countries, particularly the USA, refers to contact shortwave diathermy devices used in physiotherapy to relieve joint pain.

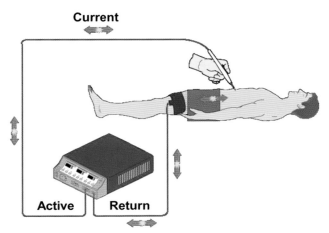

Figure 57. Monopolar Circuit

electrode used by the surgeon and a large plate electrode placed at a site some distance from the operating field. It is the commonest electrosurgical circuit used in the operating theatre.

Bipolar currents are most often used with specifically designed forceps in which the tines are electrically isolated from each other so current flows through the patient only between the tips of the forceps (Figure 58). Bipolar currents are lower voltage than monopolar because of the lower impedance of the small volume of tissue within the circuit. Bipolar circuits are therefore safer but clinically less useful due to restricted techniques principally confined to tissue coagulation. However recent advances in bipolar technology have now led to effective cutting devices used

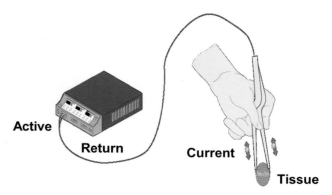

Figure 58. Bipolar Circuit

in bipolar prostatectomy and large vessel sealing devices such as *Ligasure*™ (Covidien Inc).

Frequency

Electrosurgery circuits use alternating currents (Figure 59). Mains current frequency is 60 Hz (cycles per second) and will cause electrocution and death from cardiac arrest if passed across any human even at currents as low as 1 milliamp.

Modern electrosurgical generators use alternating currents at frequencies between 200 kHz and 3.3 MHz at currents up to 2 Amps with no neuromuscular disturbance. However stimulation may occur when these currents are used close to muscle or nerve due to direct injury (galvanic stimulation) or creation of eddy currents at lower harmonic frequencies than 10 kHz (faradic stimulation; e.g. the 'obturator kick' seen in urological surgery when using electrosurgery close to the ureteric orifices).

Electrosurgical currents are either continuous or attenuated. In continuous outputs the current flow is uninterrupted but in attenuated outputs the current is broken into packets of current flow separated by a period when no current is flowing. Continuous currents are used for monopolar cutting techniques and in bipolar circuits. Attenuated currents are used for monopolar blended cutting, desiccation (coagulation), fulguration and spray techniques. Attenuated outputs are higher voltage than continuous outputs compensating for the period in which there is no current flow. In consequence as this period

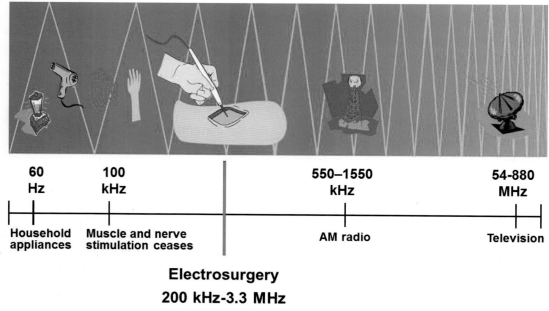

60 Hz	100 kHz		550–1550 kHz	54-880 MHz
Household appliances	Muscle and nerve stimulation ceases		AM radio	Television

Electrosurgery
200 kHz-3.3 MHz

Figure 59. The Electromagnetic Spectrum

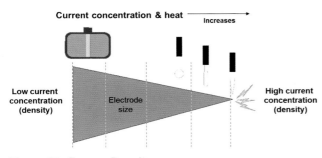

Figure 60. Energy Density

increases in outputs such as fulguration or spray the voltage is increased further.

Energy Density

The heat generated by an electrosurgical current is inversely proportional to the surface area through which it flows i.e. the smaller the surface area through which current flows the greater the heat generated. Heat can be generated along *any* part of an electrosurgical circuit if it passes through a small enough surface area. This effect is used by the surgeon with a surgical electrode e.g. forceps, blade or point, which has a small surface area and avoided in monopolar surgery at the patient plate electrode which has a large surface area[2]. This physical phenomenon of electrosurgical circuits is called energy density (also current or power density) (Figure 60).

Electromagnetic Induction

All electrical circuits generate a magnetic field perpendicular to the flow of electrons. Alternating electrosurgical currents generate magnetic fields of alternating polarity which lie in the AM radio band (Figure. 59) and can be picked up as noise on a radio playing in the operating theatre. This has led to the term radiofrequency surgery or radiofrequency current being used for these circuits. This electromagnetic phenomenon is not used clinically by the surgeon but

can be a source of unwanted burn injury when current is induced by capacitance in tissue or instruments placed close to the current path.

Adhesive gel pad electrodes have no metal to tissue contact and conduct electricity by capacitance.

Monopolar Surgical Techniques

There are four basic surgical techniques available to the surgeon when using monopolar electrosurgery; pure cutting, blended cutting, desiccation and fulguration. Pure cutting and blended cutting are products of the yellow switch on the electrosurgical generator and desiccation and fulguration of the blue switch[3].

Each technique depends upon

- The output chosen by the surgeon on the electrosurgical generator.
- The shape of the electrode used by the surgeon
- How the surgeon applies the electrical current to the patient

Cutting

Pure cutting is used infrequently in surgery as there is little haemostasis in this technique. It is used to minimise lateral heat damage when cutting and creates an area of necrosis only slightly greater than a scalpel (Figure 61).

To create a cut, the (pure) cut setting is used on the generator which is supplied using the yellow pedal or button on a finger switch electrode. This delivers a continuous alternating output (Figure. 62) to the patient. The best electrode is one which delivers a high energy density such as a point, the narrow edge of a blade or a

---

[2] Patient plates are designed by industry standards to deliver less than 2.5 Watts / cm[2]

[3] There is no real reason why we have two sides to modern electrosurgical generators; Cut (yellow) and Coagulation (blue) except that it refers back to the switches on historic generators which generated a cut current with one coil of wire and a coagulation current with another. A blend switch was then used to combine these. Modern generators use computer chips to generate the electrosurgical current but retain the convenience of two switches and some of the original terminology.

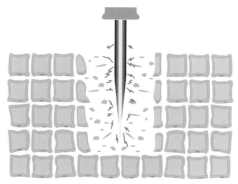

Figure 61. Cut

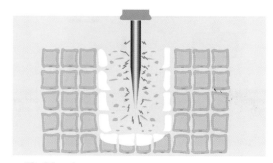

Figure 63. Blend

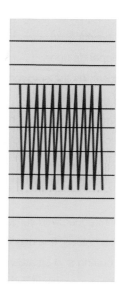

**Pure cut
(bipolar)**

Figure. 62. Cut and bipolar waveform

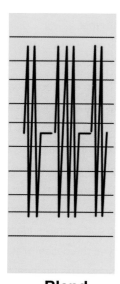

**Blend
Dessication**

Figure 64. Blended Cut Wave Form

laparoscopic hook. It is important to press the pedal before contact is made with the tissue (open circuit) and approach the tissue slowly so that small sparks (micro-sparks) can be delivered to the tissue. These sparks cause rapid boiling of cellular water, bursting the cells and creating a cleavage plane. The technique is facilitated by placing tension across the wound so that the electrode does not contact the tissue thereby losing the effects of the sparks. A faster cut can be created if the power is increased and a finer point

electrode is used. However the surgeon must be careful not to overshoot into other tissue.

Blended Cutting

Blended cut is used when small vessel haemostasis is required as the cut is created (Figure 63). The surgical electrodes and technique used is identical to pure cut. The only difference is supplied by the generator in the form of an attenuated output (Figure. 64) when the blend setting is selected. The lateral thermal spread is slightly greater than pure cut. Some generators will allow surgeons to increase

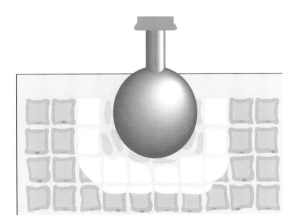

Figure 65. Desiccation

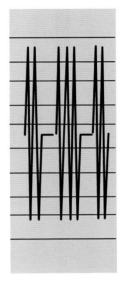

Desiccation

Figure 66. Desiccation Waveform

the degree of haemostasis (and therefore lateral thermal spread) with increasing blend settings.

Desiccation

Desiccation (contact coagulation or soft desiccation) is used to obtain haemostasis in small blood vessels (Figure. 65). This is a function of the blue switch on the generator. The appropriate setting delivers an attenuated output[4] (Figure. 66) which is applied to tissue after grasping it or applying the surgical electrode against the vessel. Lower energy density instruments are used e.g. forceps, the flat of a blade or ball electrode[5]. The heating effect obtained with this technique dries and denatures the tissue to a coagulum which seals the vessel (coaptation), assisted by vessel thrombosis. It is important to apply the current after grasping the vessel or sparks may be produced which cause a cutting effect. Similarly if overheating occurs from prolonged application at higher power settings, char may build up, increasing the impedance at the instrument tip, resulting in bypassing the char by sparking and creating a cutting effect. Char also tends to stick to the electrode and may pull away from the tissue on withdrawal of the instrument resulting in further

bleeding. Surgeons should keep power setting to a level which produces even desiccation without carbonising of the tissue.

Fulguration and Spray

Fulguration (non-contact coagulation) is used to dry an area of capillary bleeding. It is a product of the blue switch on the generator, and the appropriate setting delivers an attenuated output with the shortest period of current flow for each burst of electrical energy in the circuit (Figure. 67). It is therefore the setting with the highest voltages (up to 12,000 volts) and potential for unwanted effects. Any electrode shape can be used but in general a blade or point is most efficient. The circuit is activated before approaching the tissue. At approximately 1mm from the tissue large sparks (macro sparks) will pass between the electrode and the tissue. These have the effect of creating surface desiccation which does not penetrate more than the tissue surface. Fulguration is facilitated by blotting the tissue dry just prior to employing the technique. Blood vessels have lower impedance than surrounding tissue

---

[4] In fact identical to the blended cut output

[5] If a finger switch electrode is being used this current may be transmitted through forceps held by an assistant

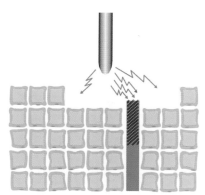

Figure 67. Fulguration

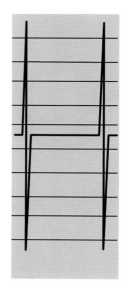

Fulguration

Figure 68. Fulguration Waveform

and will more likely attract the sparks using this technique (Figure 68).

Spray coagulation can be found on some generators and is similar to fulguration. However the voltage of the circuit is randomly varied with each spark. This has the effect that individual sparks will be attracted to different impedance tissues giving a more even effect.

Generator Sounds

The blue and yellow switches on a generator are accompanied by a tone to indicate that the circuit is active.

The pitch of this tone varies with different manufacturers. It is advisable to keep generator tones audible to ensure theatre staff can hear when the generator is activated and hazard warnings (Figure. 69). It is useful to test the alarm systems.

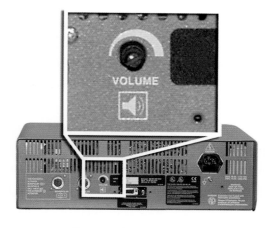

Set activation tone to audible level

Figure 69. Sound and alarm setting

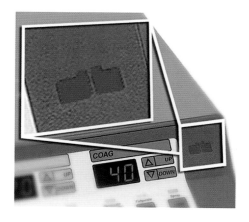

Test alarm systems

Power Setting

The surgeon should use the most appropriate power setting for the operation depending on the technique used and tissue being operated upon. Effects may vary with the greater impedance provided by some tissues, such as fat or scar, and with longer current paths where the patient plate is positioned at some distance from the operation site. In addition, different generators vary in their efficiency and require different power settings to achieve the same effect. In general the lowest power setting required to do the job should be chosen. It is therefore necessary for the surgeon to consider changing power settings on a case by case basis, or during a procedure. Fixed power settings for individual surgeons, set by protocol rather than the operation or patient should not be adhered to inflexibly.

The impedance of a monopolar circuit is significantly different in bariatric compared to paediatric patients and different power levels will be required. Similarly if the operating area and pad electrode are close to each other the impedance is lower, and lower power settings are needed. In contrast, should the surgeon find that the power setting needs to be sequentially increased in an operation whilst in the same area of dissection; it is possible that the impedance of the current path has changed and the pad electrode and connections should be checked for problems before proceeding.

Patient Plates

Most inadvertent patient burns reported to industry are due to injury under the monopolar patient plate (Figure. 70). There is a common assumption that this electrode is neutral – this is not the case. Burns do not occur under patient plates during normal usage as their size is greater than the surface area at which heating usually occurs. However any action that reduces the effective size of a patient plate will lead to burns under the plate as the energy density increases.

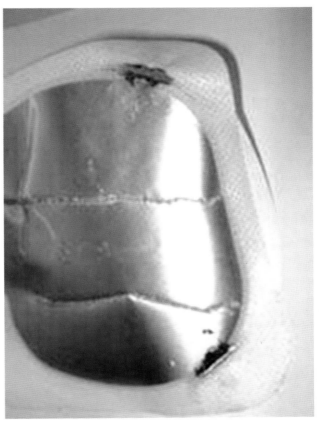

Figure 70. Pad Burns

Modern patient plate electrodes are single-use thin metal sheets of aluminium covered with an adhesive gel protected by a peel-away covering. They should be used immediately on exposing the gel and not be resealed for latter use as drying will affect the conductivity of the gel. When applied correctly these plates will provide a safe, second electrode in monopolar electrosurgery.

Older electrosurgery systems required the operating team to pre-gel plates, which were then applied with a strap; these should now be considered obsolete.

Plate positioning

In general the plate should be positioned as close to the operating field as possible to reduce the length of the current path through the patient. It should be positioned

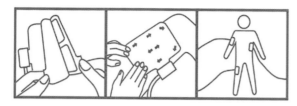

Figure 71. Pad positions

over a well vascularised, muscular area (Figure 71). The commonest position is the thigh although there is no reason why the abdomen, flank, calf or upper arm cannot be used depending on the operating site. There is no rationale for always placing it on the same thigh according to historical protocol. Some manufacturers insist that the plate is positioned with the long edge of the plate facing the operating site to avoid edge burns and this requirement should be checked prior to use. The plate should be placed with the cable in the most dependant position so it cannot peel the plate off during the operation.

It is possible to reduce the effective surface area of a patient plate and increase its current density. Areas such as bony prominences and scars present uneven impedances below the plate and should not be used as this may reduce the effective functional size of the electrode. Similarly the neck of compression stockings placed over a plate may crease the electrode and result in uneven current passage and potentiate a burn. Skin sterilising preparations can also affect the gel conductivity and should be kept away from the plate electrode. Inks in tattoos vary in conductivity and placing a plate electrode over a tattoo is probably best avoided if possible. Hair can lift a plate and hairy skin should be shaved prior to positioning.

Modern electrosurgical generators now incorporate interrogation currents that can determine if a patient plate is compromised and will alarm and turn off the main electrosurgical current under these circumstances. These plates are divided into two distinctive parts and termed split plates. The technology goes by different names depending on manufacturer (eg NESSY™ (Erbe), REM™ (Covidien Inc.))

Finally it is best to avoid using a plate position if a metal prosthesis is incorporated into the current path. Current will preferentially flow through the prosthesis due to its lower impedance and may create a heating effect where the prosthesis contacts tissue, particularly if the contact is a small surface area.

The WHO theatre checklist makes it mandatory to record whether shaving has been performed, the position of the pad electrode and the state of the skin under it following surgery. This has led to increased awareness of the possibility for electrosurgical pad burns.

Pedicle Effects

Heat generation is dependent upon the surface or cross sectional area through which the electrosurgical current is flowing. It is therefore possible in some circumstances to create a heating effect at a distance to the operating site by forcing the electrosurgical current through a narrow pedicle. Examples include ischaemic injury to the penis during circumcision or to digits during surgery on fingers and toes. Burns may occur under clips and ligatures if, for example, the cystic duct is divided or the appendix stump 'sterilised' with electrosurgery. In gynaecology tubal sterilisation with monopolar electrosurgery was abandoned due (in part) to reports of ureteric injury from current tracking. In these situations electrosurgery should be avoided unless bipolar is being used. Similarly lifting tissue away from the body e.g. the testis and using electrosurgery may create a pedicle effect and is avoided by ensuring the tissue being coagulated has broad contact with the body.

Capacitance Effects

Alternating currents generate an alternating magnetic field which spreads out perpendicular to the line of flow of electrons. Current flow may then be generated in any conductor placed within that alternating magnetic field (secondary current). This phenomenon is called capacitance.

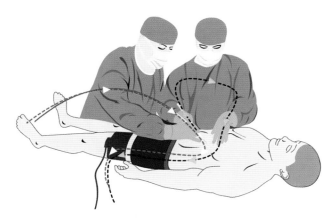

Figure 72. Assistant Glove Burn

Capacitive coupling occurs when the electrosurgical instrument lies alongside another conductor such as a metal cannula. Secondary current may then be induced in the cannula. Plastic cannulae are not entirely protective as the patient's tissue alongside a plastic cannula, or the electrosurgical instrument can itself become the secondary conductor.

Insulation failure may lead to exposure of metal in an electrosurgical instrument and inadvertent burning outside the field of view. Insulation is usually thin and instruments should be treated carefully and inspected regularly for wear and tear. Defective instruments should not be used and single-use instruments used only once.

In general, stray currents in laparoscopy are caused by a number of common factors. These include high power settings, high voltage outputs (fulguration), open circuits, long activation times and isolation of metal cannulae with a non-conducting retaining screw (hybrid cannula). The configuration of a hybrid cannula will prevent any unwanted current flow in a metal cannula from dissipating via the abdominal wall which may then pass into other structures in contact with it.

It is most easily demonstrated in relation to the electrosurgical instruments and cables (the primary conductor). Secondary currents are greatest when the two conductors lie close to each other over long lengths, with high voltage circuits (e.g. fulguration) and when this is the only pathway for current flow (open circuit). In general capacitance effects will not cause a clinical problem provided the secondary current does not discharge through a small surface area.

Clinical burns attributed to capacitance include glove burns (Figure 72), burns under towel clips used to hold cables and some laparoscopic port related burns.

Capacitance is used deliberately across a gel adhesive plate electrode.

Metal Prostheses

The metal of a prosthesis may become an internal unwanted current path if it lies between the operating site and patient return plate during monopolar electrosurgery. The metal is of lower impedance than the surrounding tissue and is taken preferentially by the circuit. This has the potential for heating and tissue damage at the narrower end of the prosthesis. Pad electrodes should therefore not be placed on the thigh of a limb with a prosthetic hip joint.

Specific Laparoscopic Issues

During laparoscopic surgery electrosurgical and other instruments are placed along cannulae into a body cavity. During surgery less than one third of the instrument may be visible to the surgeon due to the limited visual field of the laparoscope. This presents a unique surgical environment with implications for the use of electrosurgery.

Direct Coupling occurs when accidental contact is made between an active electrosurgical device and another metal instrument (cannula, laparoscope and retractor). Current may take an alternate path of less impedance along this instrument.

Jewellery

For similar reasons it is customary to tape over metal jewellery which may also become a preferential return path for the electrosurgical current giving rise to burns where the

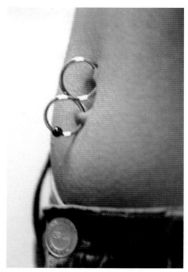

Figure 73. Jewellery

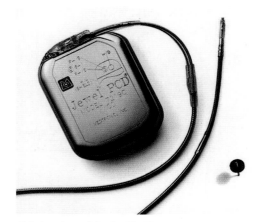

Figure 74. Implantable Defibrillator

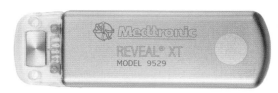

Figure 75. Implantable ECG recorder

metal touches tissue (Figure 73). Jewellery along the line of the current path should be removed.

Cardiac Devices

Implantable cardiac devices present unique problems for the patient when using monopolar electrosurgery.

Pacemakers may also become an alternate current path for the same reasons as a hip prosthesis or metal jewellery. Monopolar current passing along the pacemaker may discharge against the endocardium and change the tissue resistance to the low voltage pacing current resulting in inadequate cardiac pacing. The electronics of a pacemaker are controlled using electromagnetic induction and the magnetic field of electrosurgical cables may therefore interfere with these controls. In general it is best practice to place a pacemaker in its basic mode of demand pacing prior to surgery requiring electrosurgery. The pacemaker should not come between the operating site and the pad electrode and all cables should be routed away from the site of the pacemaker. If possible bipolar electrosurgery should be used.

Cardiac implantable defibrillators (Figure 74) detect life threatening cardiac rhythms of ventricular tachycardia or fibrillation and deliver an electrical shock to cardiovert the patient. The background electrical noise of an electrosurgical circuit is interpreted by an implantable defibrillator as ventricular fibrillation. These devices should be switched off just prior to surgery using electrosurgery and turned on again once surgery is complete.

Cardiac implantable recording devices (Figure 75) detect and store a patient's ECG over a long period and store it on its solid state chip. The electrical activity generated by an electrosurgical circuit during an operation is sufficient to fill the memory of these devices with unwanted noise. The contents of the recording device should be downloaded before and after the surgery, discarding the noise from the operation.

Generator Efficiency and Improved Safety

Modern electrosurgical generators bear little comparison to the original Bovie generator used by Harvey Cushing in 1926. Improvements have been directed in two ways; patient safety and improved surgical efficiency.

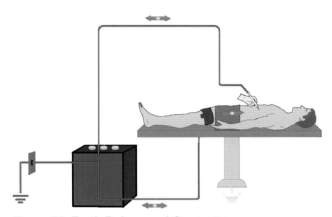

Figure 76. Earth Referenced Generator

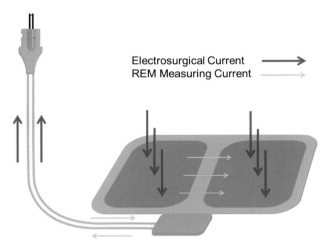

Figure 78. Pad Electrode Monitoring

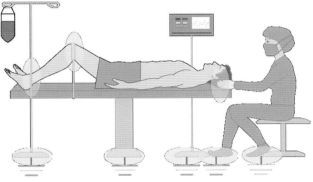

Figure 77. Leakage to Earth

Patient safety

Earth reference: Before 1970 generators were not isolated from earth (Figure 76). This meant that the electrosurgical current could leak from the patient to earth via any metal attachment or earth referenced monitor connected to the patient (Figure 77). This led to burns at these points. Modern generators create the electrosurgical current by using a transducer, isolating the electrosurgical circuit from the mains earth. The electrosurgical circuit is therefore referenced only to the generator. This has eliminated burns from leakage to earth.

Pad Technology: Modern pad electrodes are self-adhesive creating an even surface for current conduction. They are monitored by modern generators for conductivity and adhesion (Figure 78). If either changes from accepted

reference values the main electrosurgical circuit is turned off to prevent pad burns. Modern generators will also measure the impedance of the patient and limit the power of the electrosurgical circuit to prevent inadvertent burns

Surgical Efficiency

Power Output: It is generally assumed that when a generator is set to a particular setting the power is consistent across all tissue types; this is not the case (Figure 79). All generators will exhibit reduced power in higher impedance tissues such as fat and scar, reducing efficiency when dissecting these tissues. By introducing real time monitoring of the circuit voltage and current, power output can be monitored and changed to ensure constant power delivery across all clinical tissues. This is no mean feat in a circuit that changes its voltage and current up to 3 million times per second and is only available in a small number of generators. This monitoring creates a smooth and consistent effect for the surgeon during tissue dissection.

Other developments in technology include finger switches that allow the surgeon to control the power setting as well as the blue and yellow sides of the generator. Barcode labels on devices can be recognised

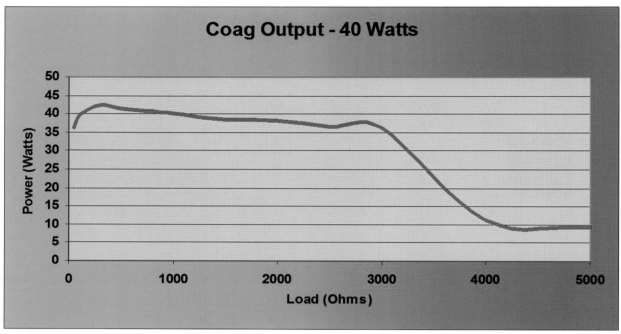

Figure 79. Power output decreasing after 3000 Ohms

by a generator and suggest optimum settings. Modern generators are driven by inbuilt software and upgrades can now be delivered by connecting the generator to a dedicated website.

Not all generators have all these features and surgeons should be involved in selecting the generator that delivers the type of technology they feel will benefit their patients during the surgery they undertake.

Ignition hazards

Hospital fires are fortunately rare. However in the operating theatre there are all the components to start a fire and care is needed to avoid this. Fires require a fuel, ignition source and an oxidiser. Fuels may be found in flammable skin preparations, drapes and plastic tubes. The sparks of an electrosurgical circuit represent an ignition source and oxygen delivered to the patient by the anaesthetist will assist combustion.

Care should be taken with all flammable substances which are placed on the patient. They should be allowed to evaporate fully before draping to prevent flammable vapour from building up in an enclosed space that can be ignited during electrosurgery. Surgery around the face and mouth should proceed after taking precautions against igniting swabs or tubes potentiated by high-dose oxygen delivered by endotracheal tube or nasal specula.

Smoke hazards

Smoke generated by burning biological tissues passes into the atmosphere of the operating theatre where it can be inhaled by staff. This applies to smoke generated by burning from any energy source, including electrosurgery.

Smoke has a particulate and a gas phase. The particles generated by burning include cellular, blood and carbon debris and vary in size. Particles in smoke from infected tissue may also include viral or bacterial debris. The gas phase is characterised by steam but also includes volatile compounds such as acrolein, benzene and toluene and small molecules such as formaldehyde, carbon monoxide and cyanide. Many of the components of smoke have

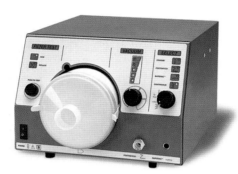

Figure 80. Smoke Evacuator

known noxious or carcinogenic effects and it would seem sensible to reduce staff exposure.

Smoke evacuation is becoming more common in operating theatres. Simple suction only removes the smoke to the suction outlet. Evacuation devices are available that filter the suctioned smoke and trap particles and contain or neutralise the chemical components (Figure 80).

Training

Studies reveal that 50% of all surgeons using electrosurgery had no training in its use. Only 20% had more than half a day's instruction. By reading this and watching the Intercollegiate Basic Surgical Skills DVD you now fall into that 30% who have had less than half a day's training in the most commonly deployed form of surgical energy used in the operating theatre. We would encourage you to continue your exploration of this subject throughout your surgical career and widen it to include an understanding of other energy sources such as argon electrosurgery, bipolar vessel sealing, harmonics and laser.

This section has been generously supported by Covidien

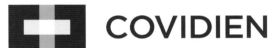

positive results for life™

Endoscopic surgery

Endoscopic surgery came of age with the development of the solid state 'chip' camera in the mid-1980s. No longer did the surgeon have to peer down a telescope and attempt surgical manipulations with one hand. The camera, held by an assistant, provided an image on a screen, leaving the surgeon free to use both hands for operative techniques, with assistants being able to view the same screen and participate effectively in the surgery. Robotic assistance is now becoming more common.

The principles of endoscopic surgery involve the closed manipulation of endoscopes and instruments while viewing a remote image (Figure 81). The operative environment is always three-dimensional, while the image is most commonly two-dimensional. These principles apply to endoscopic surgical techniques in many different specialties, from laparoscopy to thoracoscopy and arthroscopy, and from therapeutic gastrointestinal endoscopy to cystoscopic procedures. The visuospatial skills required by the endoscopic surgeon differ from those used in open surgery, and the surgeon is provided with a different set of tactile sensations than with direct manual contact.

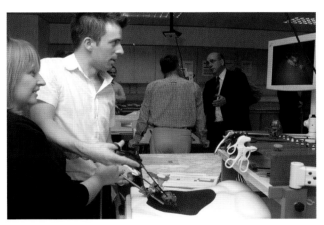

Figure 81

Depth cueing

Appropriate visuospatial awareness requires the ability to learn depth cueing of the instruments and target tissues from a two-dimensional image. The brain has many complex and interrelated mechanisms for doing this, which of course we mentally compute simultaneously. They involve the brightness of objects, perspective, assumed size, parallax and triangulation.

The brightness of objects

According to the *inverse square law* objects that are twice as close to the light source are four times brighter (Figure 82). This may be confounded if the closer object has a lighter or darker colour than the distant object.

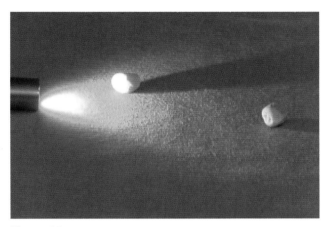

Figure 82

Perspective

Objects closer to the viewing lens appear larger than those further away, but this can be confounded by the relative size of the two objects (Figure 83).

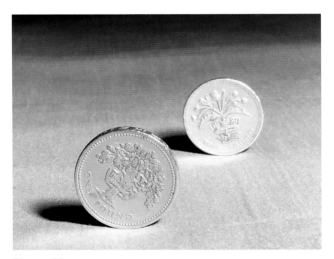

Figure 83

Assumed size

Our brains are likely to have stored information about the size of objects we have encountered or learned about. Thus if an object is known to be small but appears large in the image we assume it is close (Figure 84).

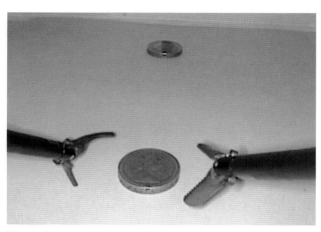

Figure 84

Parallax

A fixed movement occupies (subtends) a large angle in the visual field if it is close (Figure 85a), but only a small angle if the same movement occurs at a distance (Figure 85b).

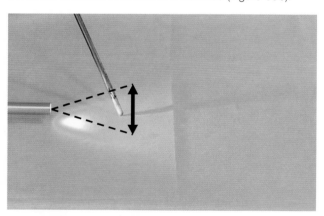

Figure 85a

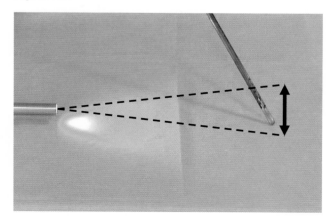

Figure 85b

Triangulation

It is difficult to judge the distance or depth of the tip of a long instrument held in one hand. However, if a second instrument is held in the other hand, then the brain can work out where the tips will meet with greater accuracy. An analogy is the principle of triangulation, which is used in navigation (Figure 86). We perform triangulation by sensing the position of all our joints in our upper limb and the length of the muscles up our arms and across our chest, together with visualisation of the instrument tips; this allows us to 'register' the position of the instruments in three-dimensional space. Once this position has been remembered the surgeon can reproduce it repeatedly, even when instruments are changed. Depending on the type of endoscopic surgery the surgeon should operate two-handed whenever possible. During a one-handed task it helps to have a second instrument safely in vision for depth cueing.

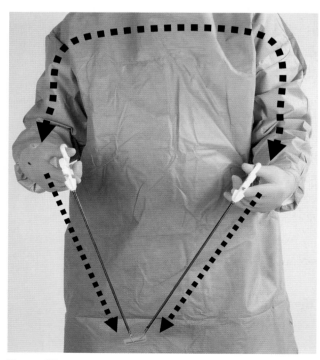

Figure 86

Fulcrum effect

When endoscopic surgery involves an instrument passing through tissues into a cavity (eg during laparoscopy, thoracoscopy and arthroscopy) the tissues act as a fulcrum or pivotal point. When the surgeon moves the instrument handle in one direction the instrument tip moves in the opposite direction (Figure 87). This is known as the *fulcrum effect*. After depth cueing it is crucial to master this and, like learning to drive on the other side of the road in another country, the time needed to master the skill is variable. According to the *law of moments*, if more than 50% of the length of an instrument passes beyond the fulcrum, then movements of the hand will produce exaggerated but less

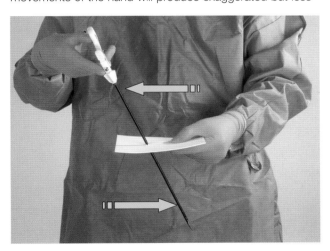

Figure 87

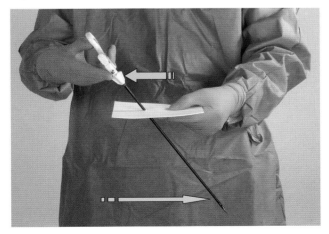

Figure 88

forceful movements of the tip (Figure 88). If less than half the instrument is beyond the fulcrum then the tip movements will be scaled down but will have greater force than the hand movements (Figure 89).

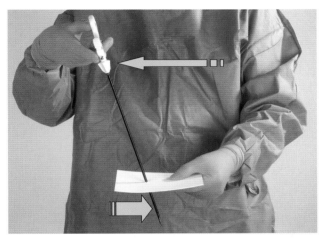

Figure 89

Camera skills

The endoscopic surgeon relies wholly on the quality and appropriateness of the image on the operating monitor. The cameraman has to master the technique of providing a stable (not rotated) image of the field of interest that the surgeon requires. Keep the site of the operative manipulations in the centre of the field of view and move with the surgeon's dissection as the procedure progresses.

A standardised set of tasks has been designed to practise depth cueing and the fulcrum effect as well as hand–eye coordination and instrument skills. Choosing appropriate instruments is important and you should remember there may be more than one way of completing the task. These tasks will be undertaken in a laparoscopic box trainer, but the skills learned are generic.

- **Peas in a pot (Figure 90):** remove the peas from the pot with a grasper (a one-handed task, but keep the other instrument in view). Then replace each pea in the pot, by first picking it up and passing it to the grasper in the other hand (a two-handed task).

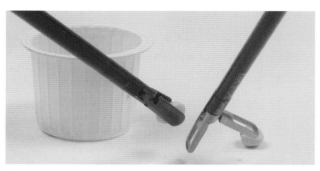

Figure 90

- **Sugar-cube stacking (Figure 91):** build a tower of sugar cubes (you may find that two instruments are needed for parts of the task).

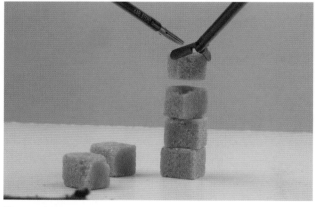

Figure 91

- **Cutting a circle from a glove (Figure 92):** cut a circle from the stretched-out rubber glove, carefully following the target circle. This involves 'roticulation'

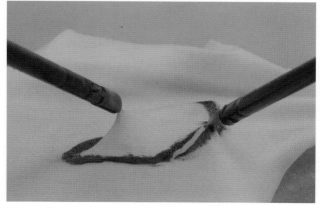

Figure 92

(the scissors may be able to be rotated by a knob on the handle) or rotation of the scissors to alter the angle of cut to achieve a more accurate circular excision. Avoid cutting the back side of the glove.

- **Mints on a string:** Thread four ring-shaped mints onto the string and tie a reef knot, all within the box trainer. Thread the mints on the string (Figure 93). There is more than one way of doing this.

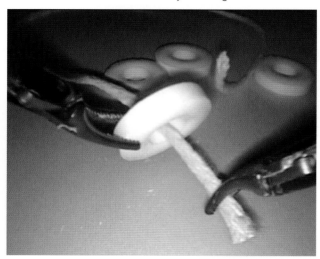

Figure 93

- **Intracorporeal reef knot:** Spend time getting the suture ends in the correct place, and the throws become easy.
- Start by forming the long end of the suture into the letter C (Figure 94).

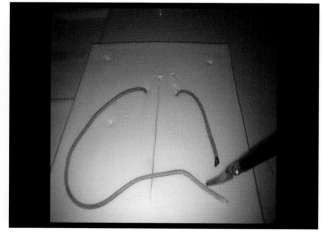

Figure 94

- Pick up the end of the long end with the opposite instrument, and rotate it so that the suture comes off the floor (Figure 95).

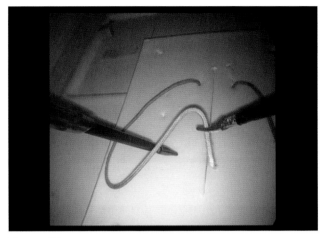

Figure 95

- Now place the other instrument over the long end and move its tip under the raised end of the long end (Figure 96).

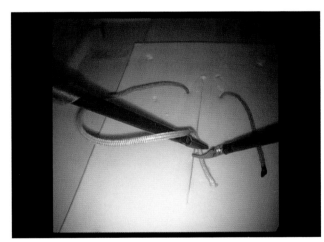

Figure 96

- Elevate the tip of this instrument so that it can pass over the tip of the other instrument and go to pick up the short end (Figure 97) to draw it through the loop by rotation rather than just pulling (Figure 98).
- Small slow movements are the key to success.

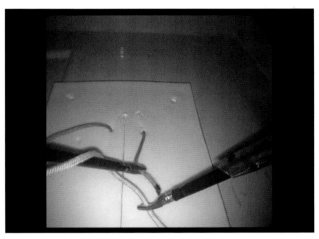

Figure 97

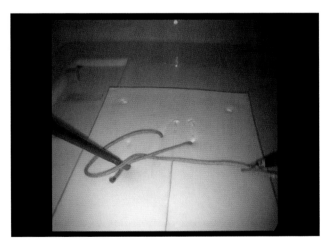

Figure 98

- Now do a reverse throw – form the reverse letter C (Figure 99) and then pick up the long end with the opposite instrument.
- Rotate the long end up (Figure 100), place the other instrument over the C, under the long end and grasp the short end (Figure 101) and draw through (Figure 102).
- This is really an instrument tie, using the left and then right hands alternately. A successful reef knot will be seen with the typical figure of eight configuration. A third throw is added by repeating the first set of movements (Figures 94-98)

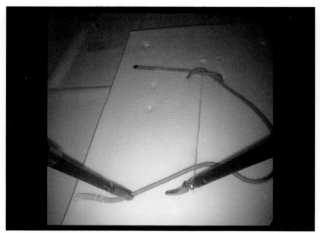

Figure 99

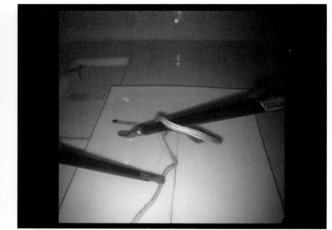

Figure 101

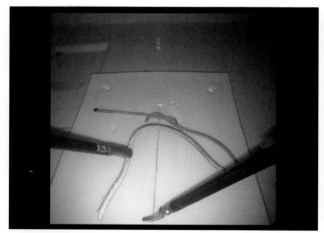

Figure 100

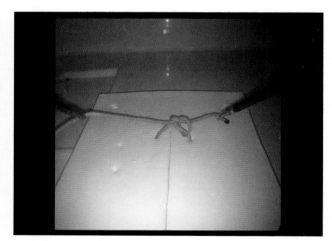

Figure 102

ASSESSMENT

Your performance will be continuously assessed throughout the course with the aim of constructing a profile of your strengths and areas for development, so that you can understand how to build on both of these. The assessments should be viewed as a way to build upon skills and improve performance in a constructive environment, rather than an ordeal to be endured.

There will be two different assessments during the course; an Objective Structured Assessment of Technical Skill (OSAT) and a continuous assessment, documented using the form found on page 66.

OSAT guidelines

The OSAT will require you to repeat one of the techniques you have been practicing during the course. Faculty will provide you with instructions and will mark you during the assessment. You will receive feedback afterwards. This assessment is intended to support your development, identifying strengths and areas for development in order for you to discuss how to improve your overall performance.

Continuous assessment guidelines

Below you will find guidelines for filling out the assessment form (Figure 103), which will be undertaken with the assistance of a faculty member at the end of each half day of the course. You will discuss the reflective section with the faculty member at your table, have a written record of areas of strength and areas for development and

will receive a score. The course director will oversee all assessments and give each participant an overall score at the end of the course. The great majority of participants are expected to satisfactorily perform during the course and will receive a certificate of completion after the course. Only participants who receive an 'unsatisfactory performance', as their overall score will need to repeat the whole 2 day course. We do not anticipate that many participants will fall into this category. It is expected that participants will demonstrate improvement over the duration of the course.

Reflective Sections

The reflective parts of the form should reflect **specific** areas within each task where you felt yourself to be particularly strong or particularly in need of improvement. You should avoid generic statements such as 'knotting', 'tendon repair' (Figure 104) and should focus on specific aspects, such as 'spacing of sutures', 'crossing hands' (Figure 105). Likewise the 'Development Plan' should consist of specific and measurable actions to take forward, rather than vague or generic statements (Figure 106). An appropriate example is given in Figure 107. Faculty members will support you by engaging with you in constructive dialogue.

Scoring and Scale

You will also be scored on a five point scale for each half day of the course. The guidelines for the scale are found on page 68.

Intercollegiate Basic Surgical Skills assessment and feedback form

Participant... Date...............................

Course...

DAY ONE AM	DAY ONE PM
Participant What aspects did I do well? What aspects would I wish to improve on next time?	**Participant** What aspects did I do well? What aspects would I wish to improve on next time?
Faculty Initials: Score: Comment:	**Faculty Initials:** Score: Comment:

DAY TWO AM	DAY TWO PM
Participant What aspects did I do well? What aspects would I wish to improve on next time?	**Participant** What aspects did I do well? What aspects would I wish to improve on next time?
Faculty Initials: Score: Comment:	**Faculty Initials:** Score: Comment:

Development Plan – How am I going to make use of the skills I have learnt?
1.

2.

Course Director Overall Comment:

Signature: **Overall Score:**   /5

Skin Suture OSAT: /17

Figure 103

```
DAY ONE AM
Participant
What aspects did I do well?

Gloving and Gowning
Knot tying
Handling Instruments

What aspects would I wish to
improve on next time?

Suturing Techniques
```

Figure 104. Poor reflective technigue

```
DAY ONE AM
Participant
What aspects did I do well?

Safe practices with sharps
Making sure I cross my hands
correctly

What aspects would I wish to
improve on next time?

Ensuring correct suture tension
Making sure sutures are spaced
correctly
```

Figure 105. Good reflective technique

```
Development Plan – How am I going to make use of the skills I
have learnt?

1. Practice knot tying

2. Doing another tendon repair
```

Figure 106. Poor reflective technique

```
Development Plan – How am I going to make use of the skills I
have learnt?

1. Making time to have a regular session in the skills lab to
practice and improve spacing of sutures

2. Simulating knot tying at home to practice and maintain
appropriate crossing of hands
```

Figure 107. Good reflective technique

5 = An **outstanding performance**, to be judged against the standard expected at completion of their stage of training

This responds to the need to highlight the fact that all participants will need to develop and improve post course as this is a basic level course. The feedback section and development plan support this. This does not therefore mean 'perfect' but means the best that can be expected taking into account level and experience. Participants who are self-aware and quick to learn may achieve this by the end of the course, particularly on the repeat exercises. It is not expected that many participants will achieve this early on in the course.

4 = A **good performance** where occasional errors are identified and corrected by the participant themselves

Participants achieving this level will show self-awareness. Small errors may be made but participants will identify, understand and demonstrate competently how to correct errors themselves.

3 = A **satisfactory performance** where occasional errors are identified by the participant, however support may be needed to correct these errors

Participants achieving this level will demonstrate self-awareness in identifying errors they may have made but may require guidance in order to correct them. They will demonstrate competence in correcting these errors, once identified.

2 = A **performance** where occasional errors are made and are not identified by the participant. Once identified by Faculty and with support, participants are able to correct errors

Participants achieving this level will not demonstrate self-awareness when they make mistakes, however they will be able correct them with appropriate guidance.

1 = An **unsatisfactory performance** with frequent errors, which raises concerns for basic safety

This score relates to the BSS assessment objectives and rationale; the course should identify the rare participant who raises concerns for basic safety. BSS is designed to develop participants and maximise the number of satisfactory completions, it is therefore expected that only a very small number of participants will achieve an unsatisfactory score.

Gloves and surgical handwashing

The choice of surgical scrub and gloves is critically important to a surgeon. This point is often not fully realised or appreciated.

Surgical handwashing

Surgical handwashing using approved scrub solutions is a technique that involves an initial washing of the hands and forearms, which removes transient micro-organisms and reduces the count of resident flora, and a second wash which further reduces the level of resident colonising flora.

Traditionally a sterile brush was used for the first application of the day, but continual use is inadvisable as damage to the skin may occur. New alcohol-based formulations have been found to be suitable for use for surgical hand scrub and for brushless application.

Alcohol antiseptics are as effective and have as wide a spectrum of antimicrobial activity as the more conventional methods using antiseptic detergent solutions and are no more damaging to the skin. Therefore, scrub solutions should be chosen that:

- have substantial initial reduction of transient and resident flora;
- are effective against a wide spectrum of micro-organisms;
- have a persistent effect and will continue to work after application (in case of glove puncture);
- are not damaging to the skin.

Hand washing technique (4 minutes)

- Adjust the water temperature, then the flow to avoid splashing.
- During washing, keep your arms in front of you with the hands higher than the elbows so the water runs down away from the hands and off at the elbows (Figure 108).

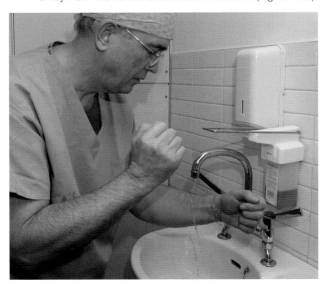

Figure 108

- Dispense the antimicrobial solution with the elbow (Figure 109).

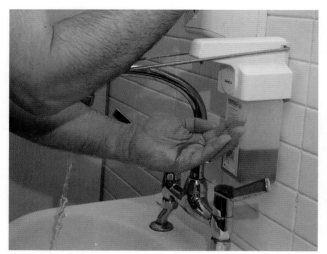

Figure 109

- Rub the hands palm to palm (Figure 110).

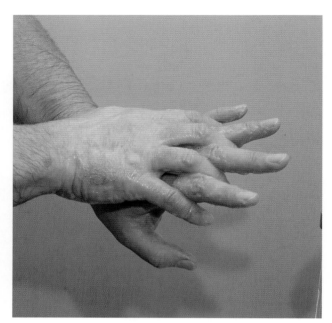

Figure 111

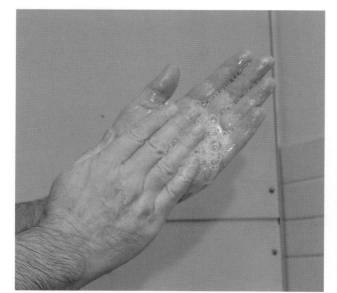

Figure 110

- Rub palm to palm with fingers interlaced (Figure 112).

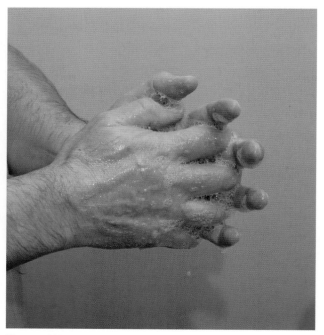

- Rub your left palm over right dorsum of hand and repeat with right palm over left dorsum (Figure 111).

Figure 112

- Rub backs of fingers with the opposing palms with the fingers interlocked (Figure 113).

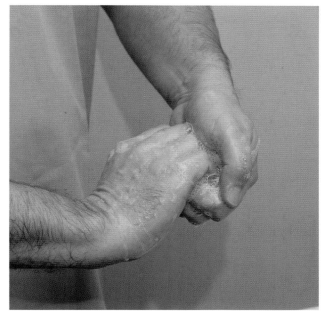

Figure 113

- Grasp the thumb with the opposing hand and rub by rotating the hand (Figure 114). Repeat with the other thumb and hand.

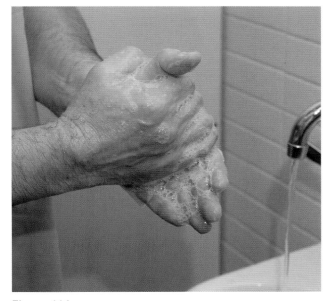

Figure 114

- Rub the palm of each hand with the clasped fingers of the opposing hand (Figure 115).

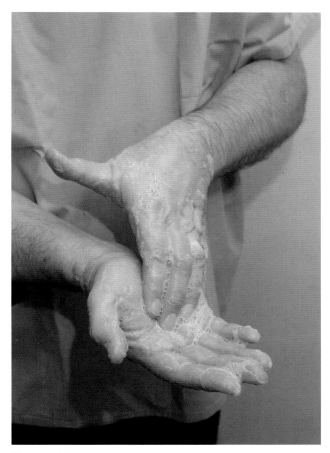

Figure 115

- Rub the left wrist and arm to within a few centimetres of the elbow using the right hand (Figure 116). Repeat for the other arm.

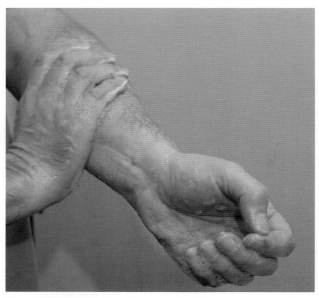

Figure 116

- If the scrub is the first of the session, brush under the nails but avoid the skin (Figure 117).

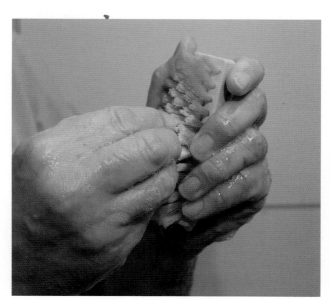

Figure 117

- Wash the forearms again but stop one third of the way from the elbow (Figure 118).

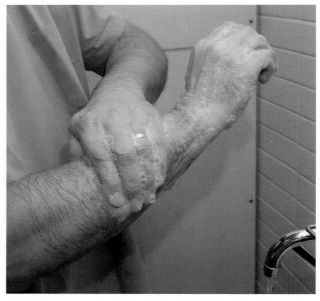

Figure 118

- Rinse the hands and arms thoroughly, keeping the hands up so the water runs down to the elbows (Figure 119).

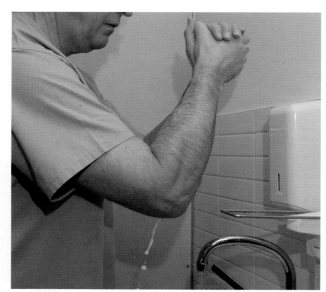

Figure 119

- At arm's length use the first towel to dry one hand and arm. Pat, not rub, the skin dry working towards the elbow (Figure 120).

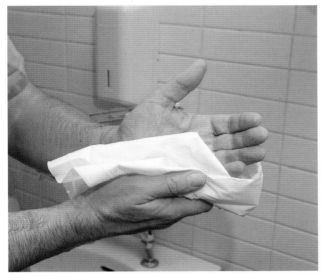

Figure 120

- Drop the towel when you reach the elbow. Repeat using the second towel for the other arm (Figure 121).

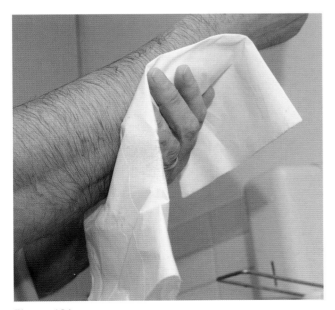

Figure 121

Choice of gloves

Given the length and complexity of many operations it is obvious that gloves must fit securely and offer optimum sensitivity and durability without causing hand fatigue. They should not lose their shape or integrity during use.

Less well understood is the need for the gloves to be of high quality, low in extractable latex proteins, and powder-free. It is well-documented that adhesions and other postoperative complications including delayed wound healing can be attributed to glove powder which transfers latex proteins from the surface of the glove.

The surface of the glove must also be low in residual accelerators used in the manufacturing process because these can cause localised skin conditions, sometimes occurring up to 48 hours after contact. With increased usage of latex gloves the incidence of latex allergy in the US has risen to between 28% and 67% in some high-risk healthcare workers and is estimated to affect 6% of the general population. Latex allergy often takes time to develop; there can be months or even years of exposure before any reaction occurs. Although latex is still recognised as the best barrier, latex-free alternatives should be considered when sensitisation occurs to the proteins in natural rubber latex.

Gloves should also be pyrogen-free, as pyrogens can induce pyrexia and misdiagnosis in some patients. This fact is also well documented.

Powder-free, latex-free synthetic gloves should also be available for:

- wearers who are known to be type 1 latex allergic (and therefore prone to anaphylactic shock);
- patients who may be at higher risk of latex allergy (such as those with spina bifida, previous atopy, dermatitis, asthma or food allergies) or those who have undergone multiple surgical procedures.

These gloves should be of the same high quality as latex gloves, allowing comfort and sensitivity, and must be part of a total protocol within a surgical unit to eliminate risk to sensitised individuals.

Glove puncture is commonplace during surgery and occurs in over 50% of cases in some operative procedures. Studies show that between 50% and 92% of perforations pass undetected. Therefore, for many procedures it would be prudent to double-glove using a green under-glove to ensure added protection. The use of two surgical gloves has been shown to maintain the barrier between the wearer and patient in four out of five cases in which the outer glove has been breached. The Biogel Reveal™ system will allow early identification of up to 97% of all glove punctures. The inner glove is a half size larger than the outer to optimise sensitivity, dexterity and comfort. If the outer glove is punctured, fluid penetrates between the two gloves and a dark green patch alerts the wearer that a puncture has occurred and the outer glove can then be replaced.

In summary, therefore a surgeon should choose a glove that:
- is suitable for the surgical procedure;
- fits well and does not lose its shape or integrity;
- offers optimum sensitivity and durability;
- is powder-free;
- contains low levels of latex allergens and residual accelerators and is pyrogen free;
- is powder-free and synthetic for those with an allergy to natural rubber latex.

Powder-free, latex-free gloves should also be available for suitable emergency cases.

This section has been generously supported by Mölnlycke Health Care.
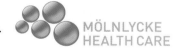

APPENDIX B

Needles

Selection of appropriate needles

Surgical eyeless needles are manufactured in a wide range of types, shapes, lengths and thicknesses. The choice of needle to be used depends on several factors such as:

- the requirements of the procedure;
- the nature of the tissue being sutured;
- the accessibility of the operative area;
- the gauge of suture material being used;
- the surgeon's preference.

Regardless of use, however, all surgical needles have three basic components – the point, the body and the swage (Figure 122).

The point depends on the needle type (see below). The body of the needle usually has a flattened section so that the needle can be grasped by a needle holder. In addition, some needles have longitudinal ribs on the surface that reduce rotational movement and ensure the needle is held securely in the jaws of the needle holder. If the needle does not have a flattened section it should be grasped at a point approximately one-third of its length away from the butt (Figure 123).

The majority of surgical needles nowadays are eyeless; that is, they are already swaged to the suture material. The many advantages of this include reduced handling

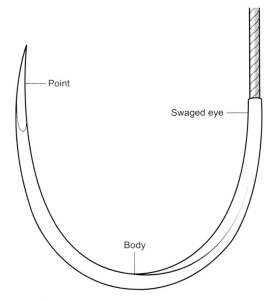

Figure 122

and preparation and less trauma to the tissue (a needle with an eye needs to carry a double strand which creates a larger hole and causes greater disruption to the tissue). A swaged (eyeless) needle has either a drilled hole or a channel at the end for insertion of suture material. The hole or channel is closed round the suture material in the swaging process.

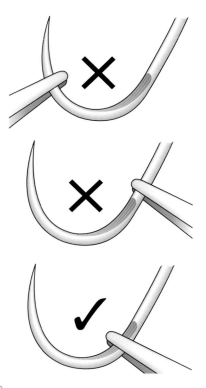

Types of surgical needles

Needles are normally classified according to needle type. The main categories are described here.

Round-bodied needles

These are designed to separate tissue fibres rather than cut them and are used either for soft tissue or in situations where easy splitting of tissue fibres is possible. After the passage of the needle the tissue closes tightly around the suture material, so forming a leak-proof suture line that is particularly important in intestinal and cardiovascular surgery.

Figure 123

Needle type	Description	Typical applications
Intestinal	The hole made by this needle is no larger than the diameter of the needle. The hole is then filled by the suture material, so reducing risk of leakage	Gastrointestinal tract; biliary tract; dura; peritoneum; urogenital tract; vessels; nerve
Heavy	In certain situations particularly strong needles with a large diameter are required	Muscle; subcutaneous fat; fascia; pedicles
Blunt taperpoint	Needlestick injury is a major concern, particularly in the presence of blood borne viruses. The blunt taperpoint is designed to prevent accidental glove puncture	Uterus; pedicles; muscle; fascia
Blunt point	This was designed for suturing extremely friable vascular tissue.	Liver; spleen; kidney; uterus; cervix

Cutting needles

Cutting needles are required where tough or dense tissue needs to be sutured.

Needle type	Description	Typical applications
Tapercut	This combines the initial penetration of a cutting needle with the minimal trauma of a round-bodied needle. The cutting tip is limited to the point of the needle, which tapers out to merge smoothly into a round cross-section	Fascia; ligament; uterus; scar tissue
Cutting	This has a triangular cross-section with the apex on the inside of the needle curvature. The effective cutting edges are restricted to the front section of the needle	Skin; ligament; nasal cavity; tendon; oral
Reverse cutting	The body of this needle is triangular in cross-section with the apex on the outside of the needle curvature	Skin; fascia; ligament; nasal cavity; tendon; oral

In addition, there are surgical needles for specialist areas, such as microsurgery, ophthalmics and endoscopic surgery.

Needle shape

The choice of needle shape is frequently governed by the accessibility of the tissue to be sutured. Normally, the more confined the operative site, the greater the curvature required. The following table shows the basic shapes and typical applications.

Shape		Typical application
Straight	————————	Skin; subcuticular; purse-string
1/4 circle		Eye; microsurgical fascia; muscle; vascular; plastic; skin; subcuticular
3/8 circle		Eye; fascia; muscle; vascular; plastic; skin; subcuticular
1/2 circle		Gastrointestinal tract; pelvis; respiratory tract; peritoneum; muscle; urogenital tract
5/8 circle		Urogenital tract; pelvis; oral cavity
J-shape		Laparotomy closure; vagina; rectum (per anus)
Compound curve		Oral; eye, anterior segment

This section has been generously supported by Ethicon Limited. **ETHICON**

APPENDIX C

Suture materials

Characteristics of suture

'The ideal suture would consist of material that permits its use in any operation, the only variable being the size as determined by the tensile strength. It should handle comfortably and naturally to the surgeon. The tissue reaction stimulated should be minimal and should not create a situation favourable to bacterial growth. The breaking strength should be high in small calibre. A knot should hold securely without fraying or cutting. The material must be sterile. It should not shrink in tissues. It should be non-electrolytic, non-capillary, non-allergenic and non-carcinogenic. Finally, after most operations the suture material should be absorbed with minimal tissue reaction after it has served its purpose.'

Postlethwait RW. *Wound Healing in Surgery.* Somerville, NJ: Ethicon Inc., 1971, pp. 8–9.

No single type of suture material has all these properties and, therefore, no suture material is suitable for all purposes. The requirement for wound support varies in different tissues from a few days for muscle, subcutaneous tissue and skin, to weeks or months for fascia and tendon, and to long-term stability for vascular prostheses.

However, the surgeon must be assured that the selected suture has the following properties:

- predictable performance;
- pliable for ease of handling and security of knots;
- minimal tissue reaction;
- high uniform tensile strength, permitting use of finer sizes;
- sterile, ready for use;
- consistently uniform diameter per size.

Types of suture materials

Suture materials are either absorbable or non-absorbable.

Absorbable sutures offer temporary wound support over a period of time and thereafter are gradually absorbed, either through a process of enzymatic reaction (catgut) or hydrolysis (synthetic material). It is important to recognise that losing tensile strength and losing mass absorption are

Suture	Type	Raw material	Tensile strength retention	Mass absorption rate	Contraindications	Frequent uses
Glycolide and lactide	Absorbable braided, coated	Copolymer of lactide and glycolide coated with polyglactin 370 and calcium stearate	28 days	56–70 days	Being absorbable, should not be used where prolonged approximation of tissues under stress is required	Ligate or suture tissues where absorbable material is desirable except where approximation under stress is required; ophthalmology
Glycolide and lactide (rapid absorption)	Absorbable braided, coated	Copolymer of lactide and glycolide coated with polyglactin 370 and calcium stearate	10–14 days	42 days	Should not be used in tissues that heal slowly and require support beyond 7 days	For closure of skin and mucosa, eg minor surgery, paediatric surgery, perineal repair, oral mucosa, scalp wounds, wounds under plaster
Glycolide	Absorbable braided, coated	Polymer of glycolic acid	30 days	60–90 days	Being absorbable, should not be used where prolonged approximation of tissues under stress is required	Ligate or suture tissues where absorbable material is desirable except where approximation under stress is required
Polydioxanone	Absorbable monofilament	Man-made polymer	56 days	180 days	Being absorbable, should not be used where prolonged approximation of tissues under stress is required	Abdominal and thoracic closure; subcutaneous tissue; colon and rectal surgery
Poliglecaprone	Absorbable monofilament	Copolymer of glycolide and caprolactone	21 days	90–120 days	Should not be used in neural tissue, cardiovascular, microsurgery, ophthalmology (except strabismus) or where extended support is required	Subcuticular skin suturing; ligation; gastrointestinal; muscle

Suture	Type	Raw material	Tensile strength retention	Mass absorption rate	Contraindications	Frequent uses
Silk	Non-absorbable braided	Natural protein fibre of raw silk spun by silk worm	Loses most or all in about 1 year	Usually cannot be found after about 2 years	Should not be used for placement of vascular prostheses or artificial heart valves	Most body tissues for ligation and suturing; general surgery; ophthalmology
Polyester	Non-absorbable braided	Man-made	Indefinite	Non-absorbable; remains encapsulated in body tissues	None	Cardiovascular; general surgery; retention e.g. drains
Braided polyamide	Non-absorbable braided	Polyamide polymer	Loses 15–20% per year	Degrades at a rate of 15–20% per year	None	Most body tissues for ligating and suturing; general closure; neurosurgery
Monofilament polyamide	Non-absorbable monofilament	Polyamide polymer	Loses 15–20% per year	Degrades at a rate of 15–20% per year	None	Skin closure; retention; plastic surgery; ophthalmology
Polyproplyene	Non-absorbable monofilament	Polymer of propylene	Indefinite	Non-absorbable; remains encapsulated in body tissues	None	General; plastic; cardiovascular; skin closure; ophthalmology

This section has been generously supported by ETHICON. ETHICON

two separate events. A suture may support the wound for only a very short time and yet may be present as a foreign body for a long period after. The ideal suture is one that would disappear immediately after its work was complete, but such a suture does not yet exist.

Non-absorbable sutures do not absorb, but some, especially those of biological origin, lose strength without any change in the mass of the suture material. Others gradually fragment over time. Yet other non-absorbables, especially those of synthetic origin, never lose tensile strength or change in mass following implantation.

Sutures can be subdivided into monofilament or multifilament. A monofilament suture is made of a single strand; it resists harbouring micro-organisms and ties down smoothly. Although monofilament sutures may tie smoothly,

they often do not lie down well, and are not nearly so secure. A multifilament suture consists of several filaments twisted or braided together, giving it good handling and tying qualities.

A further classification is based on the origin of the raw material – either biological or man-made. Sutures have been produced from a biological or natural source for many thousands of years; they tend to create greater tissue reaction than man-made sutures, sometimes resulting in localised irritation or even rejection, and have another disadvantage whereby certain patient factors, such as infection and general health, can affect the rate at which enzymes attack and break them down. On the other hand, man-made or synthetic sutures are very predictable and elicit minimal tissue reaction.

APPENDIX D

Wound management

Definition
'A wound may be defined as the loss of continuity of epithelium, with or without loss of underlying connective tissue (ie muscle, bone, nerves) following injury.' (Leaper *et al*, 1998).

'This is an injury to the skin or underlying tissues/ organs caused by surgery, a blow, a cut, chemicals, heat/cold, friction/shear force, pressure or as a result of disease, such as leg ulcers or carcinomas.' (Bale, 1997).

Principles of wound healing

Accurate assessment and treatment of the wound is dependant on:

- an understanding of the physiology of healing;
- an understanding of the factors that can affect wound healing; and
- an understanding of the optimum conditions required to maximise wound healing.

Inappropriate wound management often occurs as a result of either the inability of practitioners to correctly identify the stage of healing or differentiate between normal and abnormal characteristics associated (Flanagan, 1996).

Wound healing and classification

The wound healing process is one of repair, where damaged tissue is restored by the formation of connective tissue and re-growth of epithelium (Tortora and Gradowski, 1996). Healing is by primary (suturing) or secondary intention.

However, we must remember that wound healing is a continuous biological process so there is some overlap between phases and a sound knowledge of the structure and function of the skin is key.

Wounds can be classified into three types: superficial, dermal and full thickness.

Superficial

The exposed nature of the epidermis ensures it is often subject to trauma from physical and chemical stimuli. Common types of wounds include abrasions and first or second degree burns. Epidermal wound healing is by regeneration and is usually complete within 24–48 hours.

Dermal

When tissue damage extends through to the dermis, the process of wound healing follows through three principle stages:

- inflammation;
- proliferation; and
- maturation.

Inflammatory phase

The inflammatory phase can be subdivided into two phases: early and late.

Following initial wounding, the wound haemorrhages, platelets are activated, blood clotting occurs and the result is haemostasis, created by the formation of a platelet haemostatic plug formation and the formation and maintenance of fibrin.

Late inflammation

This is the body's natural response to injury and is characterised by the clinical signs:

- erythema;
- heat;
- oedema/discomfort; and
- functional disturbance (Tortora and Gradowski, 1996).

Inflammation

Inflammation is part of the normal protective response by the body to injury and although clinical signs are similar to those of infection, they should *not* be confused as being so. Patients who are immunosuppressed are unable to produce a typical inflammatory response and may therefore fail to activate the normal healing process (Baxter, 1994).

Wound exudate

Wound exudate is developed during this stage due to the increased permeability of the capillary membranes. It bathes the wound with nutrients and actively cleanses the wound's surface from debris including necrotic/sloughy tissue, a process known as autolysis. It is also a growth medium for phagocytic cells (Katz *et al*, 1991) such as neutrophils and macrophages. Excessive production of exudate can occur here and this can lead to skin maceration and skin sensitivities if not managed. Inflammatory exudate contains plasma proteins, antibodies, erythrocytes and white blood cells, nutrients, growth factors and enzymes.

Proliferation

During this phase the wound is filled with new connective tissue and a decrease in wound size is achieved by a combination of the three main processes:

- granulation;
- contraction; and
- epithelialisation (Flanagan, 1999).

Maturation phase

This final phase begins approximately 20 days after injury and may continue for up to a year or longer (Clark, 1988). Complete healing is when the epithelial cells have completely bridged the surface of the wound. Remodelling of scar tissue involves the type III collagen laid down during proliferation being replaced by type I collagen and there is extensive reorganisation. As remodelling occurs the cellular activity reduces and the number of blood vessels in the repair decreases (Centre for Medical Education, 1992).

The moist wound healing theory

The normal physiological process of wound repair is 'dry healing', the formation of a scab. However, the principle of moist wound healing, discovered by George Winter (1962), showed through a study carried out on pigs that epithelialisation occurred at twice the rate in moist wounds, covered by film dressings, compared to those kept dry by exposure. It is well documented that collagen synthesis and dermal repair is faster in a moist environment also (Alvarez et al, 1983; Dyson et al, 1988). Moist wound healing can be achieved with advanced wound care dressings: hydrofiber, hydrocolloid, hydrogels and films. Moist wound healing is not suitable for all wounds, such as necrotic digits, as a result of ischaemia and neuropathic, neuro/ischaemic diabetic ulcers.

Factors affecting healing

Consideration of all intrinsic and extrinsic factors is essential during a wound assessment and will ensure faster, effective healing. Such factors include:

- age;
- social environment;
- psychological perspective;
- disease processes;
- medication;
- nutrition;
- wound infection; and
- pain.

Wound infection

Wound infection prolongs the inflammatory phase of healing and can cause distress and discomfort for the patient (White et al, 2001). The outcome depends upon the interaction of complex host and microbial factors (Emmerson, 1998).

For wound infection to develop, the following wound factors are taken into consideration: size, position, duration, local perfusion, host immunocompetency. These factors are balanced against number and type of invading microbial species (microbial bioburden) and the presence of foreign bodies, including necrotic tissue and eschar (White et al, 2001).

The mere presence of bacteria should not automatically indicate a clinical diagnosis of wound infection. There are four documented stages along the infection continuum (Ayton, 1985):

- *Contamination* of a wound refers to bacteria, which are present but not multiplying in the wound bed.
- *Colonisation* refers to the presence of multiplying bacteria which are not causing a host reaction.
- *Critical colonisation* is the state at which the multiplying bacteria are causing the wound to move in favour of the bacteria and are starting to cause a host reaction. Such subtle indicators include an alteration in pain and sensation in the wound bed, a non-healing wound, presence of thick slough and an intransigent odour.

- *Wound infection* is defined as the presence of multiplying pathogenic bacteria, which are causing a host reaction.

Several signs and symptoms accompany wound infection but not all wounds exhibit these at any one time. Such signs and symptoms include:

- pain, heat, erythema, cellulitis;
- pyrexia;
- malodour;
- oedema to wound margins;
- pathogenic bacteria (confirmed by a wound swab);
- delayed healing/wound breakdown; and
- fragile granulation tissue which bleeds easily.

Treatment should be based upon achieving a host-manageable bioburden (Bowler, 2003). 'Silent infections' can occur, especially in patients who are immunocompromised or have certain metabolic disorders, ie diabetes, so the presence of a non-healing wound should make the practitioner consider the presence of infection also.

References

Alvarez OM, Mertz PM, Eaglstein WH. The effect of occlusive dressings on collagen synthesis and re-epithelialisation in superficial wounds. *J Surg Res* 1983; **35**: 142–148.

Ayton M. Wounds that won't heal. *Nursing Times (Community Outlook)* 1985; **81**: 16–19.

Bale S, Jones V. *Wound Care Nursing: a patient-centred approach*. London: Bailliere Tindall; 1997.

Baxter CR. Immunologic reactions in chronic wounds. *Am J Surg* 1994; **167(1A)**: 12S–14S.

Bowler PG. The 105 bacterial growth guideline: reassessing its clinical relevance in wound healing. *Ostomy Wound Manage* 2003; **49**: 44–53.

Centre for Medical Education. *The Wound Programme*. Dundee: University of Dundee; 1992.

Clark RAF. Overview and general consideration of wound repair. In: Clark RAF. *The Molecular and Cellular Biology of Wound Repair*. New York: Plenum; 1988.

Wound Care Society. Wound swab procedure. *Journal of Wound Care* 1993; **2**: 77.

Dyson M *et al*. Comparison of the effects of moist and dry conditions on dermal repair. *J Invest Dermatol* 1988; **91**: 435–439.

Emmerson M. A microbiologist's view of factors contributing to infection. *New Horiz* 1998; **6 (2 Suppl)**: S3–10.

Flanagan M. A practical framework for wound assessment 1: physiology. *Br J Nurs* 1996; **5**: 1,391–1,397.

Flanagan M. The physiology of wound healing. In: Miller M, Glover D. *Wound Management: Theory and Practice*. London: Nursing Times Books; 1999.

Katz MH *et al*. Human wound fluid from acute wounds stimulates fibroblasts and endothelial cell growth. *J Am Acad Dermatol* 1991; **25**: 1,054–1,058.

Leaper DJ, Gottrup F. Surgical wounds. In: Leaper DJ, Harding KG. *Wounds Biology and Management*. Oxford: Oxford University Press; 1998. pp 23.

Lewis B. Nutrition and age in the aetiology of pressure sores. *J Wound Care* 1997; **6**: 41–42.

Moore P, Foster L. Acute surgical wound care 1: an overview of treatment. In: White R, Harding K. *Trends in Wound Care*. London: Mark Allen Publishing; 2002.

Moy SL. Wound healing. *Management of Acute Wounds* 1993; **11**: 759–760.

Tortora GJ, Gradowski SR. *Principles of Anatomy and Physiology*. 7th ed. Hoboken, New Jersey: Wiley; 1996.

White RJ, Cooper R, Kingsley A. Wound colonization and infection: the role of topical antimicrobials. *Br J Nurs* 2001; **10**: 563–578.

Williams NJ, Leaper DJ. Infection. In: Leaper DJ, Harding KG. *Wounds: Biology and Management*. Oxford: Oxford University Press; 1998.

This section has been generously supported by ConvaTec. ConvaTec A Bristol-Myers Squibb Company

APPENDIX E

Evaluation

Online Surgical Course Participant Evaluation (SCOPE)

Participant Guide

Your evaluation as a participant is an essential part of maintaining the quality and directing development of the Royal College of Surgeons of England courses in an aim to improving surgical standards across the country.

The online evaluation form consists of three main parts:

1. Demographic questions;
2. Generic questions appropriate to all courses (e.g. your experience of enrolment through to overall satisfaction).
3. Course specific questions reflecting how successfully the course achieved its intended learning outcomes. These are followed by opportunities to add more detail to your feedback through 'free text' boxes.

The evaluation is stored and analysed anonymously and names are used only to check and validate responses

Evaluations are an integral requirement of the course and as such you should complete the online evaluation as soon as possible after the course whilst your memory is fresh, or at the latest within 2 weeks of completion of the course.

TO COMPLETE YOUR ONLINE EVALUATION:

Enter via the direct web-link: http://survey.rcseng.ac.uk/wix1/p632700610.aspx

Or through the Course Evaluation link on the Education page of the Royal College of Surgeons website: http://www.rcseng.ac.uk/

It should take no more than 10 minutes to complete.

As the online evaluation marks the final part of the course attendance, certificates from your course can only be issued once feedback has been received. Unfortunately if after 4 weeks you have not submitted your feedback, you will not be automatically certificated and you will need to order a copy via the RCSENG website: this will incur an administration fee.

http://www.rcseng.ac.uk/education/order-your-certificate

Thank you for taking the time to evaluate your course, your opinion matters to us and will help to inform future course planning, if you have further comments or require an individual reply, please email the Education inbox Education@rcseng.ac.uk.

Acknowledgements

Membership of the Intercollegiate Working Party for the Fifth Edition

Bill Thomas (Chairman)

Rory McCloy (The Royal College of Surgeons of England)

David Smith (The Royal College of Surgeons of Edinburgh)

Brian Lane (The Royal College of Surgeons in Ireland)

Paul Teenan (The Royal College of Physicians and Surgeons of Glasgow)

Louise Goldring (The Royal College of Surgeons of England)

The Royal College of Surgeons of England Basic Surgical Skills Steering Group

Rory McCloy (Chairman)

Bill Thomas

Christopher Backhouse

Nick Gillham

David Monk

John Weston Underwood

Louise Goldring

Please note

While every effort has been made to ensure the accuracy of the information contained in this publication, no guarantee can be given that in its compilation all errors and omissions have been excluded. Readers wishing to use this information are recommended therefore to verify the facts for themselves when appropriate.

Photography by the photographic studio, The Royal College of Surgeons of England.

Design by Chatland Sayer, London.

Illustrations by Oxford Designers and Illustrators Limited.

Gloving illustrations by Ben Pepper (Royal College of Surgeons of England).

Appendix A illustrations by ETHICON; Electrosurgery illustrations by Covidien.

Printed by Henry Ling Limited, Dorchester, Dorset.

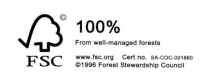

100%
From well-managed forests
www.fsc.org   Cert no. SA-COC-001860
©1996 Forest Stewardship Council

08.15 WIMAT Cardiff Medicentre Heath Park CF14

Wednesday 7th October   4UJ

Day 1

08.15 - 08.30	Registration	* Park on Level 3 only.
08.30 - 08.40	Introductions	
08.40 - 9.00	Gowning + gloving	VP 041
9.00 - 09.50	Knots -	VP 042

One handed reef
Instrumental tie

09.50 - 10.50   Surgeons knot
Tying at depth

11.05 - 11.30   Handling instruments
Scissors, haemostats, forceps, scapel

11.30 - 13.00   Suturing techniques
Interrupted.
Simple
Mattress
Continuous
Subcuticular

13.45 - 1455   Ligation / transfixion
Pedicle transfixion
Continuity tie
Pedicle tie

14.55 - 15.55   Tissue Handling 1
Bowel:- End-end interrupted
(hand tied knots - no assistance)

16.10 - 16.55   Tissue Handling 2
Tendon repair - assisted

17.10 - 17.30   Discussion + feedback